Frontiers of Neurology and Neuroscience

Vol. 27

Series Editor

J. Bogousslavsky   *Montreux*

Neurological Disorders in Famous Artists – Part 3

Volume Editors

J. Bogousslavsky   *Montreux*
M.G. Hennerici   *Mannheim*
H. Bäzner   *Stuttgart*
C. Bassetti   *Lugano*

62 figures, 19 in color, and 8 tables, 2010

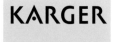

Basel · Freiburg · Paris · London · New York · Bangalore ·
Bangkok · Shanghai · Singapore · Tokyo · Sydney

·······················
Frontiers of Neurology and Neuroscience
Vols. 1–18 were published as Monographs in Clinical Neuroscience

Julien Bogousslavsky, MD
Center for Brain and Nervous System
Disorders, and Neurorehabilitation
Services
Genolier Swiss Medical Network
Clinique Valmont
CH-1823 Glion/Montreux (Switzerland)

Michael G. Hennerici, MD
Department of Neurology
University of Heidelberg
Universitätsmedizin Mannheim UMM
Theodor-Kutzer-Ufer 1-3
DE-68167 Mannheim (Germany)

Claudio Bassetti, MD
Neurocenter of Southern Switzerland
Department of Neurology
Ospedale Civico
Via Tesserete 46
CH-6903 Lugano (Switzerland)

Hansjörg Bäzner, MD
Department of Neurology
Klinikum Stuttgart, Bürgerhospital
Tunzhofer Strasse 14-16
DE-70191 Stuttgart (Germany)

(As requested by the Library of Congress, CIP data for Part 1 (vol. 19) are printed).
Library of Congress Cataloging-in-Publication Data

Neurological disorders in famous artists / volume editors, J. Bogousslavsky,
F. Boller.
    p. ; cm. – (Frontiers of neurology and neuroscience ; v. 19)
  Includes bibliographical references and index.
  ISBN 3-8055-7914-4 (hardcover : alk. paper)
  1. Nervous system–Diseases. 2. Artists–Diseases
  [DNLM: 1. Famous Persons–Case Reports. 2. Nervous System Diseases–Case
Reports.] I. Bogousslavsky, Julien. II. Boller, François. III. Series.
  RC359.N46 2005
  616.8–dc22

                        2005002444

Bibliographic Indices. This publication is listed in bibliographic services, including Current Contents® and
Index Medicus.

© Copyright 2010 by S. Karger AG, P.O. Box, CH–4009 Basel (Switzerland)
www.karger.com
Printed in Switzerland on acid-free and non-aging paper (ISO 9706) by Reinhardt Druck, Basel
ISSN 1660–4431
ISBN 978–3–8055–9330–4
e-ISBN 978–3–8055–9331–1

Contents

Preface

This is the third volume of 'Neurological Disorders in Famous Artists', a 'series' we initiated in 2005 highlighting the relationship between neurological disease and creativity in famous painters, writers, poets, philosophers, and musicians. The first trigger was the important observation that the biographic reports of Guillaume Apollinaire available at that time failed to match the actual changes in his personality and activity after World War I, mainly because of unwarranted psychological interpretations in a man who in fact suffered from a traumatic brain lesion, with subsequent paralysis, epilepsy, and associated emotional behaviors. Following this landmark several examples of dramatic modifications in artistic output after stroke, brain tumor or other neurological diseases were identified in poets such as Guy de Maupassant, painters like Caspar David Friedrich and Anton Räderscheidt, or composers including George Gershwin, Joseph Haydn or Maurice Ravel, which we addressed in the preceding volumes. On the other hand, we also emphasized that neurological diseases can sometimes be the start of artistic renewal, as was the case in Willem de Kooning (dementia), Carl Fredrik Reuterswärdt or Lovis Corinth (stroke). In this third volume, we present a series of painters, musicians and writers who also had to fight against an acute or chronic neurological disease, sometimes without success (e.g. Shostakovich, Schumann, Wolf, and Pascal), but often with a dynamic and paradoxically creative integration of the clinical disorder into their artistic production (e.g. Klee and Ramuz). The case of Blaise Cendrars is particularly striking; he lost his right writing hand during the war in 1915 and developed phantom pain which considerably influenced his subsequent work, written with the left hand. Forty years later he lost the use of his left hand after a stroke; he partly recovered, but was finally paralyzed after stroke recurrence. Writers may also occasionally write the first report of a medical condition that they observed in themselves. This was the case for Stendhal who made the first detailed report of aphasic transient ischemic attacks, before he died of a stroke shortly thereafter. In other, fortunately rarer instances, a neurological disease has been inaccurately attributed to an artist in order to explain certain features of his work, the best example being de Chirico whose paintings supposedly were influenced by migraine or epilepsy from which he is unlikely to have suffered. Egon Schiele's depiction of his body in self-portraits rather displayed emotions and psychic conflicts in dystonia-like poses he knew from photographs of hysterical patients, but he did not himself suffer from the disease. Similarly in this volume some chapters focus on neurological conditions reported in artistic work. We already know about hemiplegia or chorea in Egyptian frescoes, and of the Babinski sign in baby Jesus' foot being kissed in medieval paintings, but less known are certain conditions described by Shakespeare, Dumas, and in operas.

The editors are grateful to the erudite authors of the chapters herein, often striking and entertaining, and which bring new light to both artists and neurological conditions.

Julien Bogousslavsky
Michael G. Hennerici
Hansjörg Bäzner
Claudio Bassetti

Bogousslavsky J, Hennerici MG, Bäzner H, Bassetti C (eds): Neurological Disorders in Famous Artists – Part 3. Front Neurol Neurosci. Basel, Karger, 2010, vol 27, pp 1–10

· ·

Leonardo da Vinci and Stroke – Vegetarian Diet as a Possible Cause

Şerefnur Öztürk[a], *Marta Altieri*[b], *Pina Troisi*[b]

[a]Department of Neurology, Ankara Numune Education and Research Hospital, Ankara, Turkey, and [b]Department of Neurological Sciences, Clinica Neurologica A, 'Sapienza' University of Rome, Rome, Italy

Abstract

Leonardo da Vinci (April 15, 1452 to May 2, 1519) was an Italian Renaissance architect, musician, anatomist, inventor, engineer, sculptor, geometer, and painter. It has been gleaned from the many available historical documents that da Vinci was a vegetarian who respected and loved animals, and that he suffered from right hemiparesis in the last 5 years of his life. A vegetarian diet has both positive and negative influences on the cerebrovascular system. In this report, a possible relation between a vegetarian diet and stroke is discussed from various perspectives as related to Leonardo da Vinci's stroke.

Copyright © 2010 S. Karger AG, Basel

Leonardo da Vinci: As a Vegetarian Artist

Leonardo da Vinci (born April 15, 1452 in Vinci; died May 2, 1519 in Ambroise) was an Italian Renaissance architect, musician, anatomist, inventor, engineer, sculptor, geometer, and painter (fig. 1) [http://www.settemuse.it]. He has been described as the archetype of 'Renaissance man' and a universal genius. Da Vinci is famous for his masterly paintings, among them 'The Last Supper' and 'Mona Lisa', and is also known for his designs and inventions, many of which anticipated modern technology, though few of them were constructed in his lifetime. In addition, he helped advance the study of anatomy, astronomy, and civil engineering [http://www.artinvest2000.com; http://www.leonardo2007.com; http://www.bilanciozero.net; http://www.centroarte.com; http//italian.classic-literature.co.uk/leonardo-da-vinci].

The first known biography of da Vinci was published in 1550 by Giorgio Vasari in his 'Vite de' piu eccelenti architettori, pittori e scultori italiani' ('The

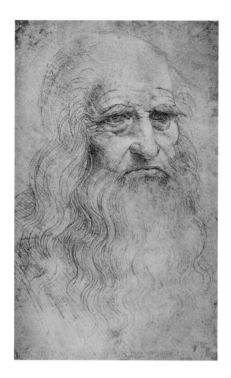

Fig. 1. Portrait of Leonardo da Vinci. With kind permission from the Ministerio per i Beni e le Attività Culturali, Biblioteca Reale, Turin, Italy.

lives of the most excellent Italian architects, painters and sculptors'). Most of the information collected by Vasari was from first-hand accounts of da Vinci's contemporaries, and remains the preeminent reference in studying da Vinci's life [http//italian.classic-literature.co.uk/leonardo-da-vinci].

Born the illegitimate son of a notary, Piero da Vinci, and a peasant woman, Caterina, at Vinci in the region of Florence, Leonardo was a man of universal genius and talent, who fully embodied the spirit of the Italian Renaissance, leading to higher forms of expression in various fields of art and knowledge. As a painter, sculptor, architect, engineer, anatomist, writer, musician and inventor, he is considered one of the greatest geniuses of mankind.

Leonardo has often been described as a man whose unquenchable curiosity was equaled only by his powers of invention [Richter, 1977]. He is widely considered to be one of the greatest painters of all time and perhaps the most diversely talented person ever to have lived [http://manybooks.net/pages/davincietex-t048ldvc10/0.html]. According to art historian Helen Gardner [1975], the scope and depth of his interests were without precedent, and 'his mind and personality seem to us superhuman, the man himself mysterious and remote' [Richter, 1977].

The personality of Leonardo da Vinci was always surrounded by an aura of mystery. He was sometimes not accepted and often closed out by ideology.

Aside from his artistic nature, Leonardo possessed highly unique and interesting personal features. It is known that he was a vegetarian who respected and loved animals [http//italian.classic-literature.co.uk/leonardo-da-vinci].

We have glimpses into his lifestyle from his own writings and from what was written about him by the early biographers. Da Vinci's refusal to eat animals and his recognition of the cruelty of their mistreatment have been referenced. Jean Paul Richter was historically the first person to decipher Leonardo's notebooks. In his epochal 'The Literary Works of Leonardo da Vinci' [Richter, 1977] he wrote:

> 'We are led to believe that Leonardo himself was a vegetarian from the following interesting passage in the first of Andrea Corsali's letters to Giuliano de'Medici: "Alcuni gentili chiamati Guzzarati non si cibano dicosa alcuna che tenga sangue, ne fra essi loro consentono che si noccia adalcuna cosa animata, come it nostro Leonardo da Vinci". ("Certain infidels called Guzzarati [Hindus] do not feed upon anything that contains blood, nor do they permit among them any injury be done to any living thing, like our Leonardo da Vinci").' Giuliano de'Medici, incidentally, was a patron of da Vinci and the brother of Pope Leo X.

Eugene Muntz [1898] wrote, 'It appears from Corsali's letter that Leonardo ate no meat, but lived entirely on vegetables, thus forestalling modern vegetarians by several centuries'.

In 'The Mind of Leonardo da Vinci' (1928), Edward MacCurdy wrote:

> '…Vasari tells, as an instance of his love of animals, how in Florence when he passed places where birds were sold he would frequently take them from their cages with his own hand, and having paid the sellers the price that was asked would let them fly away in the air, thus giving them back their liberty.'

In 'Leonardo: Discovering the Life of Leonardo da Vinci' Bramly [1991] wrote: 'Leonardo loved animals so much, it seems, that he turned vegetarian'. Da Vinci was also referred to as a vegetarian in 'Leonardo da Vinci – The Mind of The Renaissance' by Alessandro Vezzosi [1997], founder and director of the Museo Ideale Leonardo da Vinci in Vinci, Italy [http://www.ivu.org].

Leonardo da Vinci: As a Stroke Victim

It has been ascertained from many documents that Leonardo da Vinci suffered from right hemiparesis in the last 5 years of his life. Vezzosi [1997] stated that the semi-paralysis of the right side of da Vinci's body would not have affected the left-handed artist's ability to sketch, but did hamper his mobility: 'It probably prevented him from standing up to paint and from holding a palette – but he would still have had enough strength to sit down and draw'. He further writes: 'The painting shows us an elderly Leonardo with all the signs of age, with his right hand sus-

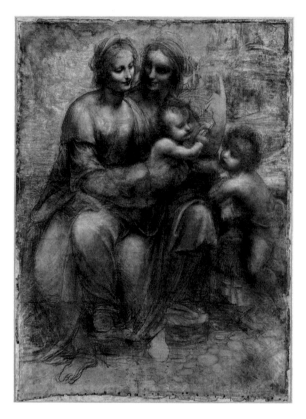

Fig. 2. Leonardo da Vinci, The Virgin and Child with the Infant John the Baptist and St. Anne. The Leonardo Cartoon (about 1499–1500). © The National Gallery, London.

pended in a stiff, contracted position, held up by his robe as if it were a bandage'. Vezzosi [1997] also reported that the paralysis would explain da Vinci's inactivity for the last 5 years of his life, with several of his paintings left incomplete.

Although suffering from a paralysis of the right hand, Leonardo continued to draw and teach. He produced studies of the Virgin Mary from 'The Virgin and Child with St. Anne' (fig. 2); studies of cats, horses, dragons, St. George, and on the nature of water; anatomical studies; and drawings of the Deluge and of various machines.

All historical sources tell us that Leonardo da Vinci used his right hand when creating all his artwork. There is no indication that he was left-handed. However, he was better with his left hand than the normal right-handed person. For example, da Vinci sometimes wrote his documents in mirror-writing with his left hand, though he never painted with his left hand! The main historical reference in this regard is from Antonio de' Beatis, secretary of the Cardinal Luigi d'Aragona, who, together with his master, paid a visit to Leonardo da Vinci on October 10, 1517. Luckily for all historians he habitually wrote down everything, quite literally, in his diary:

'On the 10th of October 1517, Monsignor (the Cardinal Luigi d'Aragona) and the rest of us went to see, in one of the outlying parts of Amboise, Messer Leonardo da Vinci the Florentine… the most eminent painter of our time, who showed to his Eminence the Cardinal three pictures: one of a certain Florentine lady (Pacificia Brandano or Isabella Gualanda), painted from life, at the insistence of the late Giuliano de'Medici; the other of the youthful St. John the Baptist; and the third of the Madonna and the Child in the lap of St. Anne, the most perfect of them all. One cannot indeed expect any more good work from him, as a certain paralysis has crippled his right hand. But he has a pupil, a Milanese, who works well enough. And although Messer Leonardo can no longer paint with the sweetness which was peculiar to him, he can still design and instruct others…' [Goldscheider, 1944].

The death of Leonardo has been described only by Vasari. He describes an old and tired man, worn out by numerous ailments. At the same time also refers to an 'evil' that plagued Leonardo and all the problems associated with this. Then he informs us of how he died and he speaks of a 'paroxysm' as a 'messenger of death'. This term should be construed as an exacerbation of his illness. Leonardo was suddenly seized by a strange illness and death occurred in a sudden and almost unexpected manner while he was talking to his illustrious visitor, the King of France. He was placed on his bed and died in the arms of the king. From such a description one would most likely imagine that a vascular event affected the great Italian genius. One can clearly infer the nature of this event, cardiac or cerebral. Vasari writes:

'Finalmente venuto vecchio, stette molti mesi ammalato, e vedendosi vicino alla morte si voles diligentemente informare delle cose cattoliche e della buona e santa religione cristiana, e poi con molti pianti confesso e contrito, sebbene e' non poteva reggersi in piedi, sostenendosi nelle braccia di suoi amici e servi, volle divotamente pigliare lo Santissimo Sacramento fuor del letto…contando il mal suo e gli accidenti di quello, mostrava tuttavia quanto avea offeso Dio e gli uomini del mondo, non avendo operato nell'arte come si conveniva. Onde gli venne un parosismo messaggiero della morte, per la qual cosa rizzatosi il re e presogli la testa per aiutarlo e porgergli favore, acciocché il male lo alleggerisse, lo spirito suo che divinissimo era, conoscendo non potere avere maggior onore, spirò in braccio a quell re nell'età sua d'anni settantacinque' [http://biblio.signum.sns.it/cgi-bin/vasari/Vasari-all? code_f=print_page&work=le_vite&volume_n=4&page_n=36].

Benefits of Vegetarianism versus Risks of Cerebrovascular Disease

Segasothy and Phillips [1999] reviewed the beneficial and adverse effects of vegetarian diets in various conditions. The vegetarian diet, which includes fruits, vegetables, complex carbohydrates, soy bean, legumes, nuts and soluble fiber, could lower the risk of cardiovascular disease through multiple mechanisms such as lowering cholesterol and the beneficial effect of antioxidant vitamins, folic acid, linolenic acid and fiber [Segasothy and Phillips, 1999].

Some studies have reported the beneficial effect of a vegetarian diet with respect to vascular diseases. A vegetarian diet with comprehensive lifestyle changes for 1 year showed significant overall regression in coronary atherosclerosis [Gould et al., 1992]. An inverse association between fruit and vegetable consumption and stroke has been suggested. In a population-based longitudinal study of 832 middle-aged men with over 20 years of follow-up, for each increment of three servings of fruits and vegetables per day, there was a 22% decrease in the risk of all stroke [Gillman et al., 1995].

From another perspective, however, a vegetarian diet can be seen to have some adverse effects, and there may in fact be a relation between a vegetarian diet and stroke. For example, while a vegetarian diet can be useful for a short duration, its effects over the long term must be argued as contributing to stroke risk. Adverse effects of a vegetarian diet include the following: while most vegetables oils are low in saturated fatty acids, some are rich in them, and a high intake is associated with elevated plasma cholesterol levels and may be associated with atherosclerosis [Council on Scientific Affairs, 1990]. The Nutrition Committee of the American Heart Association concluded that trans fatty acid has adverse effects on cholesterol profiles [Lichtenstein, 1997].

It has been shown that vegetarians have a higher risk of stroke since their intake of total fat and saturated fat is low, and their serum cholesterol level is low [Segasothy and Phillips, 1999]. As a possible mechanism, it has been suggested that low-fat vegan diets tend to downregulate systemic insulin-like growth factor (IGF)-I activity, which acts on vascular endothelium to activate nitric oxide synthase, thereby promoting vascular health; this downregulation of IGF could thus be expected to increase stroke risk in vegans [McCarty, 2003].

In addition, there is important proof showing a relationship between a vegetarian diet and levels of vitamin B_{12}, folic acid and homocysteine. Substantial nutritional deficiencies in these three vitamins along with mild hyperhomocysteinemia, perhaps through an interplay with the classical cardiovascular risk factors (highly prevalent in this population), could further aggravate the risk of coronary artery disease [Iqbal et al., 2005]. The intake of vitamin B_{12} is lower in vegetarian diets and deficiencies in this vitamin have been reported in vegetarians, especially in vegans, and this deficiency leads to an increase in plasma homocysteine concentration [Abdulla et al., 1981; Huang et al., 2003; Sanders et al., 1978].

In one study, homocysteine values and lipid parameters were measured in groups of adults consuming alternative nutrition (vegetarians/lacto-ovo/vegans) and compared with a group consuming traditional diets (omnivores, general population). The frequency of hyperhomocysteinemia was 53% in vegans and 28% in vegetarians vs. 5% in omnivores. It was concluded that low lipid risk factors but higher findings of mild hyperhomocysteinemia in vegetarians indicated a diminished protective effect of alternative nutrition in cardiovascular disease prevention [Krajcovicová-Kudláčková et al., 2000].

In a study in an elderly population investigating the relation between homocysteine blood concentrations and vitamin intake, the predominant cause of elevated homocysteine blood concentrations was inadequate blood folate [Selhub et al., 1995]. In the study by Hung et al. [2002] on the effects of a lacto-vegetarian diet on vitamin B status and plasma homocysteine level, fasting plasma homocysteine was inversely correlated with plasma folate and vitamin B_{12} in the vegetarian group. Multiple regression analysis revealed that plasma folate, vitamin B_{12} and creatinine were independent determinants of homocysteine variation and contributed to 38.6% of homocysteine variation in the vegetarian versus omnivore group. In addition, fasting plasma homocysteine in the vegetarians correlated negatively with serum threonine, lysine, histidine, arginine and cysteine, and these amino acids contributed to 38.7% of homocysteine variation. It was concluded that a lacto-vegetarian diet is associated with mildly elevated fasting plasma homocysteine levels presumably due to lower levels of plasma vitamin B_{12} [Hung et al., 2002].

Hyperhomocysteinemia is accepted as an important risk factor of stroke. Elevated plasma total homocysteine is a strong, graded, independent risk factor of stroke, myocardial infarction, and other vascular events [Spence et al., 2005]. The relation between hyperhomocysteinemia and a vegetarian diet seems important and may show an aspect of the vegetarian diet and stroke risk relationship. In patients with non-valvular atrial fibrillation hospitalized for cardiac reasons, increased fasting total plasma homocysteine levels were independently associated with a history of ischemic stroke [Loffredo et al., 2005].

In a retrospective cohort study of 5,056 men and women aged 35–79 years, there was a 69% increased risk of coronary mortality among those with the lowest quartile compared with the highest quartile of serum folate [Morrison et al., 1996]. Results from the Nurses' Health Study demonstrated a significant inverse relation between a dietary intake of folate and vitamin B_6 and mortality from cardiovascular disease during a 14-year follow-up of 80,082 women [Rimm et al., 1998].

Studies have shown that high plasma homocysteine concentrations and low concentrations of folate and vitamin B_6 are associated with extracranial carotid artery stenosis and an increase in the risk of stroke [Perry et al., 1996; Selhub et al., 1993]. A total homocysteine level of >10.2 μmol/l is associated with a doubling of vascular risk, and a total homocysteine level of >20 μmol/l is associated with an 8-fold increase in vascular risk [Graham et al., 1997; Nygord et al., 1997].

Folic acid supplementation has been shown to be highly effective in reducing plasma homocysteine levels [Bouchey et al., 1995]. Supplementation with folic acid, pyridoxine and vitamin B_{12} is associated with regression of atherosclerotic plaque in the carotid artery [Peterson and Spence, 1998]. It has been suggested that an increase in folic acid and reduction in homocysteine level would potentially prevent an important number of deaths from vascular causes [Bouchey et al., 1995]. Each 100-μg/day increase in folate is associated with a 5.8% lower risk of coronary heart disease [Rimm et al., 1998].

The mechanisms by which homocysteine may cause vascular disease include a propensity for thrombosis and impaired thrombolysis [Nishinaga and Shinada, 1994; Simioni, 1999] and increased oxidation of low-density lipoprotein and lipoprotein(a) [Leerink et al., 1994]. Vitamin therapy with folate, pyridoxine (B_6), and cobalamine (B_{12}) reduces the total homocysteine level and reverses endothelial dysfunction induced by high total homocysteine [Brattström, 1996; Chambers et al., 1998; Van den Berg et al., 1994]. To decrease the homocysteine level, B_{12}, betaine, and thiols must be used together [Spence et al., 2005].

Conclusion

Leonardo da Vinci may have suffered from the adverse effects of his vegetarian diet [Ozturk, 2009]. His stroke, which resulted in right hemiparesis, may have been related to an increase in homocysteine level because of the long duration of his vegetarian diet. We are not aware of any indication suggesting a cardiac cause or of any other major stroke risk factor. Leonardo da Vinci, regarded as the archetypal universal genius, could perhaps have continued to build upon his collection of masterful works had he not suffered from limiting paresis.

References

Abdulla M, Andersen I, Asp N-G, Berthelsen K, Birkhed D, Dencker I, et al: Nutrient intake and health status of vegans. Chemical analysis of diet using duplicate portion sampling technique. Am J Clin Nutr 1981;34:2464–2477.
Bouchey CJ, Beresford SAA, Omenn GS, Motulsky AG: A quantitative assessment of plasma homocysteine as a risk factor for vascular disease. JAMA 1995;274:1049–1057.
Bramly S: Leonardo: Discovering the Life of Leonardo da Vinci (Reynolds S: English translation). Staten Island, Brainiac Books, 1991.
Brattström LE: Vitamins as homocysteine-lowering agents. J Nutr 1996;126:51276–51280.

Chambers JC, McGregor A, Jean-Marie J, Kooner JS: Acute hyperhomocysteinemia and endothelial dysfunction. Lancet 1998;351:36–37.

Council on Scientific Affairs: Saturated fatty acids in vegetable oils. JAMA 1990;263:693–695.

Gardner H: Gardner's Art through the Ages, ed 11. Boston, Wadsworth, 1975.

Gillman MW, Cupples LA, Gagnon D, Posner BM, Ellison RC, Castelli WP, et al: Protective effect of fruits and vegetables on development of stroke in men. JAMA 1995;723:113–117.

Goldscheider L: Leonardo da Vinci, ed 2. London, Phaidon Press, 1944, p 20.

Gould KL, Omish D, Kirkeeide R, Brown S, Stuart Y, Buchi M, et al: Improved stenosis geometry by quantitative coronary arteriography after vigorous risk factor modification. Am J Cardiol 1992;69:845–853.

Graham IM, Daly LE, Refsum HM, Robinson K, Brattstrom LE, Ueland PM, et al: Plasma homocysteine as a risk factor for vascular disease. The European Concerted Action Project. JAMA 1997;277:1775–1781.

Huang YC, Chang SJ, Chiu YT, Chang HH, Cheng CH: The status of plasma homocysteine and related B-vitamins in healthy young vegetarians and nonvegetarians. Eur J Nutr 2003;42:84–90.

Hung CJ, Huang PC, Lu SC, Li YH, Huang HB, Lin BF, et al: Plasma homocysteine levels in Taiwanese vegetarians are higher than those of omnivores. J Nutr 2002;132:152–158.

Iqbal MP, Ishaq M, Kazmi KA, Yousuf FA, Mehboobali N, Ali SA, et al: Role of vitamins B_6, B_{12} and folic acid on hyperhomocysteinemia in a Pakistani population of patients with acute myocardial infarction. Nutr Metab Cardiovasc Dis 2005;15:100–108.

Krajcovicová-Kudlácková M, Blazícek P, Babinská K, Kopcová J, Klvanová J, Béderová A, et al: Traditional and alternative nutrition–levels of homocysteine and lipid parameters in adults. Scand J Clin Lab Invest 2000;60:657–664.

Leerink CB, van Ham AD, Heeres A, Duif PH, Bouma BN, von Rijn HJ: Sulfhydryl compounds influence immunoreactivity, structure, and functional aspects of lipoprotein(a). Thromb Res 1994;74:219–232.

Lichtenstein AH: Trans fatty acids, plasma lipid levels and risk of developing cardiovascular disease: a statement for health care professionals from the American Heart Association. Circulation 1997;95:2588–2590.

Loffredo L, Violi F, Fimognari FL, Cangemi R, Sbrighi PS, Sampietro F, et al: The association between hyperhomocysteinemia and ischemic stroke in patients with non-valvular atrial fibrillation. Haematologica 2005;90:1205–1211.

McCarty MF: IGF-I activity may be a key determinant of stroke risk–a cautionary lesson for vegans. Med Hypoth 2003;61:323–334.

Morrison HI, Schaubel D, Desmeules M, Wigle DT: Serum folate and risk of fatal coronary heart disease. JAMA 1996;275:1893–1896.

Müntz E: Leonardo da Vinci, Artist, Thinker and Man of Science. London, Heinemann, 1898.

Nishinaga M, Shinada K: Heparan sulfate proteoglycan of endothelial cells; homocysteine suppresses anticoagulant active heparan sulfate in cultured endothelial cells. Rinsho Byoni 1994;42:340–345.

Nygord O, Nordehaug JE, Refsum H, Voland PM, Farstad M, Vollset SE: Plasma homocysteine levels and mortality in patients with coronary artery diseases. N Engl J Med 1997;337:230–236.

Ozturk S: Leonardo Da Vinci (1452–1519) as a stroke victim: hemiparesis a result of a vegetarian diet? J Med Biogr 2009;17:7.

Perry IJ, Refusm H, Morris RW, Ebrahim SB, Ueland PM, Shaper AG: Prospective study of serum total homocysteine concentration and risk of stroke in middle-aged British men. Lancet 1996;348:1120–1124.

Peterson JC, Spence JD: Vitamins and progression of atherosclerosis in hyper-homocysteinemia (letter). Lancet 1998;351:263.

Richter JP: The Literary Works of Leonardo da Vinci Compiled and Edited from the Original Manuscripts by Jean Paul Richter: Commentary by Carlo Pedretti. Berkeley, University of California Press, 1977.

Rimm EB, Willett WC, Hu FB, Sampson L, Colditz GA, Manson JE, et al: Folate and vitamin B_6 from diet and supplements in relation to risk of coronary heart disease among women. JAMA 1998;279:359–364.

Sanders TA, Ellis FR, Dickerson JWT: Hematological studies on vegans. Br J Nutr 1978;40:9–15.

Segasothy M, Phillips PA: Vegetarian diet: panacea for modern lifestyle diseases? QJM 1999;92:531–544.

Selhub J, Jackues PF, Boston AG, D'Agastino RB, Wilson PWF, Belanger AJ, et al: Association between plasma homocysteine concentrations and extracranial carotid artery stenosis. N Engl J Med 1995;332:286–291.

Selhub J, Jackues PF, Wilson PW, Rush D, Rosenberg IH: Vitamin status and intake as primary determinant of homocysteinemia in an elderly population. JAMA 1993;270:2693–2698.

Simioni P: The molecular genetics of familial venous thrombosis. Baillieres Best Pract Res Clin Haematol 1999;12:479–503.

Spence JD, Bang H, Chambless LE, Stampfer MJ: Vitamin Intervention for Stroke Prevention trial: an efficacy analysis. Stroke 2005;36:2404–2409.

Van den Berg M, Franken DG, Boers GH, Blom HJ, Jacobs C, Stehouwer CD, et al: Combined vitamin B_6 plus folic acid therapy in young patients with arteriosclerosis and hyperhomocysteinemia. J Vasc Surg 1994;20:933–940.

Vezzosi A: Leonardo da Vinci. The Mind of Renaissance (translated from French). New York, Abrahams, 1997.

Dr. Şerefnur Öztürk
Department of Neurology 1
Ankara Numune Education and Research Hospital
TR–06420 Ankara (Turkey)
Tel. +90 31 250 84501, Fax +90 31 243 16090, E-Mail serefnur.ozturk@noroloji.org.tr

Bogousslavsky J, Hennerici MG, Bäzner H, Bassetti C (eds): Neurological Disorders in Famous Artists – Part 3. Front Neurol Neurosci. Basel, Karger, 2010, vol 27, pp 11–28

....

Paul Klee's Illness (Systemic Sclerosis) and Artistic Transfiguration

Hans Suter

Fahrni, Switzerland

Abstract

Klee's symptoms, and the rapid progression of the illness, ending with his death after only 5 years, in all probability indicate the rarest but most serious form of scleroderma, known as diffuse systemic sclerosis. Although his skin and internal organs were heavily stricken by the illness, the artist's hands were fortunately spared. Thus he was able to draw and paint without hindrance to the end. Classified amongst diseases of the autoimmunity system, this form of sclerosis often has inexplicable causes. I believe, however, that the defamations suffered by Klee, his dismissal as professor of the Art Academy in Düsseldorf by the National Socialists, and the unintended isolation after his return to Berne were causative factors in the outbreak of the illness. Mentally and spiritually, the artist rose above his heavy bodily suffering. Constantly, his creativity remained vigorous. Although the greater part of Klee's works in his last years cannot be linked directly with his illness, careful viewing reveals a significant preoccupation with fate and illness. It is above all in his drawings, that were created like a diary, that the sorrows and troubles of the ill artist emerge: his fears, but also his hopes and finally his resignation to the illness, and his readiness for death. In undesired isolation, and in his own spiritual world, Paul Klee created with exemplary concentration, discipline and diligence a considerable number of late works, which differ from his early work and which deserve our full admiration. Reserved, quiet and kind, Paul Klee was nevertheless charismatic. And his art is poetic. Possessing a special aura, it can enchant those who surrender to it without any prejudice. Paul Klee has created an oeuvre that is unique, reflecting his character closely: a body of work that moves and stirs us by its deep humanity.

Paul Klee was born on December 18, 1879, in a suburb of Berne. His father was German and worked as a teacher of music. His mother was Swiss. In 1880 the family moved to Berne. Here, Klee went to school. After passing the matriculation examination he trained as an artist at the Academy of Arts in

Munich. In 1906 he married Lily Stumpf, a Munich pianist. In 1907 his only son, Felix, was born.

In 1920 Paul Klee was appointed as a teacher at the public Bauhaus, a University for art and design at Weimar. Among others Wassily Kandinsky worked at this famous arts institute. In 1930 Klee was appointed professor at the Academy of Arts in Düsseldorf.

In 1933 the artist, a distinguished and popular professor at the Academy of Arts in Düsseldorf, was dismissed by the National Socialists who had just come to power. His art was slandered as being 'unhealthy'. The National Socialists feared resistance and wanted to remove any academic teaching personnel who might be seen as spiritually or morally superior to them.

In December 1933 Paul Klee and his wife Lily returned to Berne. The artist called Berne his 'real hometown'. However, he was not received very warmly there. Klee's avant-garde art was understood only by a few friends, artists and art historians.

Exhibitions of his works were hardly noticed. The painter fell into an undesired isolation. Such a change from appreciation to disdain is a heavy strain on the psyche of any human being.

Soon after their return to Berne, Paul and Lily, being Germans, filed an application to obtain Swiss citizenship. At first they were granted a residence permit for 1 year only, which had to be renewed each subsequent year. After 5 years the Swiss authorities allowed the couple citizenship in principle. But first they had to apply for the cantonal and communal citizenship in Berne. The necessary bureaucratic procedure was protracted, with the artist being questioned by officials. After visiting Klee, a police official remarks in his report – referring to a painting 'Swiss landscape' of 1919 hanging on the wall – that the cows represented in it looked 'silly' – and I quote: 'Does this picture not aim plainly at what certain people call "Cow-Swiss"? ('Cow-Swiss' is a disrespectful name occasionally used in Germany for the Swiss). In spite of such foolish statements, Paul Klee in all probability would have obtained Swiss citizenship, however he died 6 years after filing his application and 6 days before the decisive meeting of the naturalization commission in Berne.

In summer 1935, one and a half years after emigrating from Germany, the artist suddenly fell ill with a violent, long-lasting and feverish bronchitis. Pneumonia and pleurisy followed, and he weakened.

Figure 1: Marked Man, 1935

The painting 'Marked Man', from the time his illness started, may be a self-portrait. Paul Klee was already heavily marked by the illness. The big black

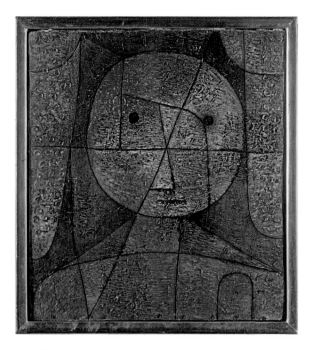

Fig. 1. Paul Klee, Marked Man, 1935, 146, oil and watercolor on primed gauze on cardboard, 32 × 29 cm. Kunstsammlung Nordrhein-Westfalen, Düsseldorf, photograph by Walter Klein, Düsseldorf, with kind permission. ©2010, ProLitteris, Zurich.

eyes look at us inquiringly and gravely. The only two lines running completely through the picture cross out the face. Significantly, the same feature appears in the painting 'Crossed from the list' from 1933. Now, however, the crossing-out may have another meaning: that the illness will end fatally.

Figure 2: Paul Klee, 1939

In 1935 changes in the skin on Klee's face and neck appeared. The skin became tense, the nose pointed and the mouth thin. His face became a 'mask-face'. His family doctor sent him for an advisory consultation to Professor Naegeli, the Professor for Dermatology at the University Hospital of Berne. It is probable that he diagnosed the condition as 'scleroderma' but, out of consideration for Klee's feelings, this was withheld from the patient.

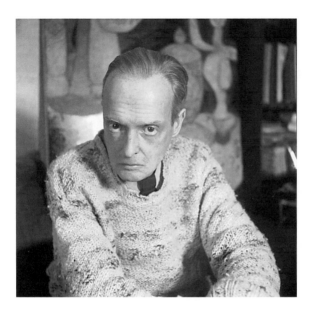

Fig. 2. Paul Klee, 1939. Photograph by Walter Henggeler. With kind permission. ©Keystone, Zurich.

Figure 3: The Eye, 1938

The painting 'The Eye' of 1938 is probably a self-portrait. The face shows the traits of a mask-face, typical of scleroderma. One eye is wide open, the other closed. The composition is in equilibrium but the represented human being is not. His condition is unstable. Klee looks thoughtfully into an uncertain future.

Figure 4: Mask: Pain, 1938

In the drawing 'Mask: Pain' of 1938 a mask-like face is deeply afflicted. The illness has progressed further. Swallowing has become painful. Klee can now consume only pulpy-liquid nourishment. This indicates a sclerodermal esophagus stenosis. Further, a stomach hemorrhage occurred and Klee developed a tendency to diarrhea and anemia. He suffered shortness of breath during physical exertion, probably as a result of lung fibrosis. The artist bore his escalating ailments with great courage.

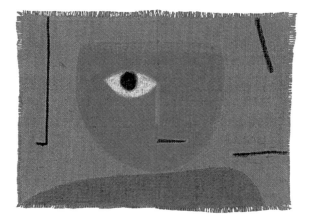

Fig. 3. Paul Klee, The Eye, 1938, 315, pastel on burlap, 45/46 × 64.5/66.5 cm. Private collection, Switzerland, on extended loan to the Zentrum Paul Klee, Berne, with kind permission. ©2010, ProLitteris, Zurich.

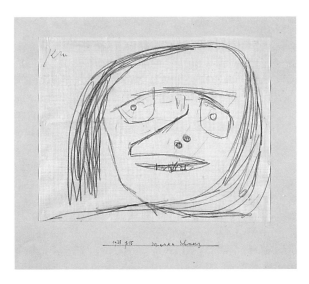

Fig. 4. Paul Klee, Mask: Pain, 1938, 235, chalk on paper on cardboard, 21 × 27.1 cm. Zentrum Paul Klee, Berne, with kind permission. ©2010, ProLitteris, Zurich.

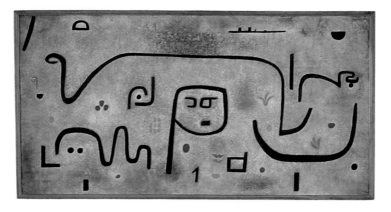

Fig. 5. Paul Klee, Insula dulcamara, 1938, 481, oil and colored paste on paper on burlap; original frame, 88 × 176 cm. Zentrum Paul Klee, Berne, with kind permission. ©2010, ProLitteris, Zurich.

Figure 5: Insula dulcamara, 1938

In 1938 the outbreak of the Second World War was imminent. Paul Klee was conscious of his privileged situation in Switzerland. He painted 'Insula dulcamara'. Dulcus (Latin) means sweet, amarus/amara bitter. He probably anticipated living on a green island, surrounded by an ocean of war, with its fear, suffering and death. The artist perceived this privilege as sweet. The central skull may be symbolic of the coming war and his personal fate which he saw as bitter. The 'bittersweet' plant, suggested in the picture, is a deadly nightshade with scarlet fruit. The National Socialists have cast their dark shadow, exiling the artist into a 'nightshade existence'!

Figure 6: Taking Leave, 1938

Two years before his death Paul Klee probably already had a premonition that his illness was incurable and that he would soon take leave. How moving this the simple picture 'Taking Leave' of 1938 is, with the serious eyes and the bowed head! Through a narrow cleft behind a dark wall he looks sadly at us. The cleft will slowly close for ever.

Klee's works from his last years drew heavily from his personal experiences and feelings. The illness progressed in steps. There were times of improvement, during which hope arose.

Figure 7: High Spirits, 1939

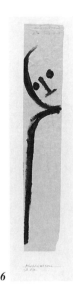

In the painting 'High Spirits' of 1939 Klee balances precariously on the tightrope. He expresses the pleasure of this successful balancing act by an exclamation mark. But how easily a slight mistake could cause the fatal fall. Paul Klee must have realized that rescue was probably not possible. The painter's novel art was not understood in Switzerland. An art critic even described his art as being schizophrenic.

Fig. 6. Paul Klee, Taking Leave, 1938, 352, colored paste on paper on cardboard, 50.7 × 7.3/9.3 cm. Zentrum Paul Klee, Berne, with kind permission. ©2010, ProLitteris, Zurich.

Fig. 7. Paul Klee, High Spirits, 1939, 1251, oil and colored paste on paper on burlap; original frame, 101 × 130 cm. Zentrum Paul Klee, Berne, with kind permission. ©2010, ProLitteris, Zurich.

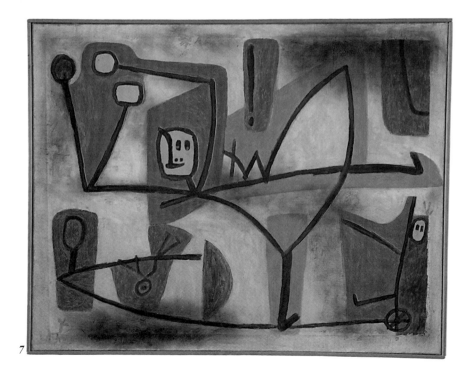

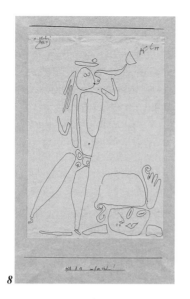
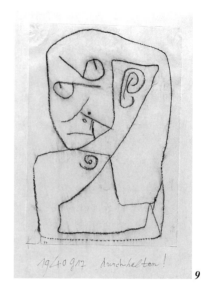

8   9

Fig. 8. Paul Klee, Rise from the Dead!, 1938, 478, pen on paper on cardboard, 29.8 × 20.9 cm. Zentrum Paul Klee, Berne, with kind permission. ©2010, ProLitteris, Zurich.

Fig. 9. Paul Klee, Stick It Out!, 1940, 337, pastel on paper on cardboard, 29.6 × 20.9 cm. Zentrum Paul Klee, Berne, with kind permission. ©2010, ProLitteris, Zurich.

Figure 8: Rise from the Dead!, 1938

The illness had greatly exhausted the artist, who doubted that any improvement was possible. In the picture 'Rise from the Dead' of 1938, parts of the body have already been detached. At the lower right-hand side we find a fallen human being. Then, however, this man stands up, stretches himself, reaches for a trumpet and blares his name out of the instrument. It is Klee himself. He gives himself courage and utters a defiant 'And yet!' against his fate.

Figure 9: Stick It Out!, 1940

A picture from the year of his death shows a meditative artist, marked heavily by his illness but still defiant, declaring vigorously that he will 'stick it out!'

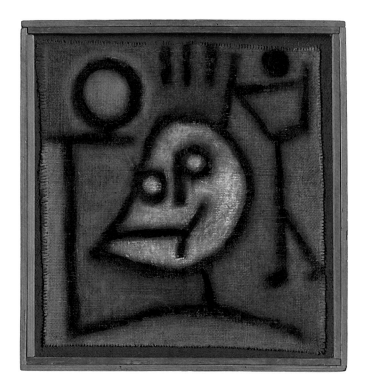

Fig. 10. Paul Klee, Death and Fire, 1940, 332, oil and colored paste on burlap; original frame, 46.7 × 44.6 cm. Zentrum Paul Klee, Berne, with kind permission. ©2010, ProLitteris, Zurich.

Figure 10: Death and Fire, 1940

In 'Death and Fire' a man leaves this world. His head is ash-grey. Mouth, nose and eyes become significant letters: 'Tod' ('death'). The head is a repetition of the scull in the painting 'Insula dulcamara' from 1938. The man's body will burn in the fire, but not the golden ball, surrounded by black, held in his upwardly stretched hand. It can be assumed that this contains the artist's lifework. It is his legacy to us. The pale, familiar face with the large eyes expresses preparedness and devotion. Paul Klee has come to terms with the unavoidable. Full of expectation, he greets us for the last time, aware of his precious legacy, which – in the form of the golden ball – he proudly holds up. It is a comforting picture, despite its sad message!

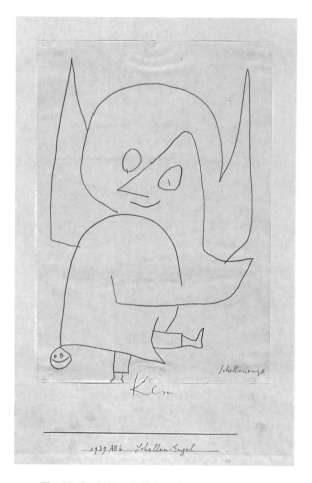

Fig. 11. Paul Klee, Bell Angel, 1939, 966, pencil on paper on cardboard, 29.5 × 21 cm. Zentrum Paul Klee, Berne, with kind permission. ©2010, ProLitteris, Zurich.

Figure 11: Bell Angel, 1939

Klee's angels are delightful angels, still half in this world albeit with one step already in the other. They show refreshingly humorous traits, reflecting Klee's love of irony.

In 'Bell Angel' the angel is tremendously pleased with the clear tinkling of a little bell hanging on the seam of his robe.

Paul Klee was a protestant, but his religiousness transcended denominations.

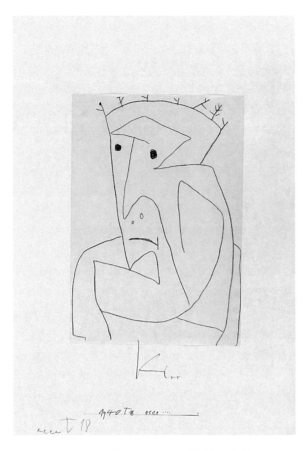

Fig. 12. Paul Klee, Ecce...., 1940, 138, chalk on paper on cardboard, 29.7 × 21.1 cm. Zentrum Paul Klee, Berne, Livia Klee Donation, with kind permission. ©2010, ProLitteris, Zurich.

Figure 12: Ecce ...., 1940

In the drawing 'Ecce ....' from the year of his death, the artist refers to the scriptural passage, where the Roman procurator Pontius Pilate presents Jesus to the people (John, 19, 5) with the declaration 'ecce homo' ('behold the man!'). Klee's reference to the scriptural passage may emerge not only from the crown of thorns, but also from the four omission points following the 'ecce', which most likely stand for the letters 'homo'. Did he draw himself as a thoughtful sufferer, who has suffered injustice and sorrow, as did Jesus?

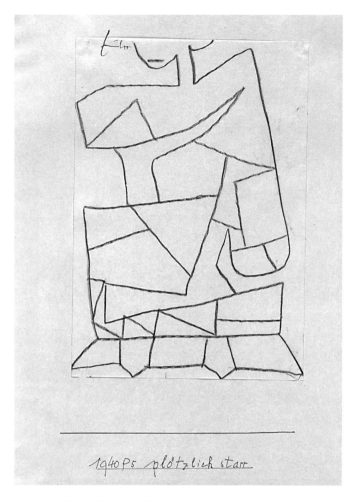

1940 Ps plötzlich starr

Fig. 13. Paul Klee, Suddenly Rigid, 1940, 205, chalk on paper on cardboard, 29.6 × 21 cm. Zentrum Paul Klee, Berne, with kind permission. ©2010, ProLitteris, Zurich.

Figure 13: Suddenly Rigid, 1940

The sclerodermal skin thickens and becomes stiff and rigid; suppleness is lost. The man in the picture – Klee himself – is shown with sharp, angular lines, denoting his inflexible, diseased skin. At the same time, Klee was stiff with horror at what was happening in Germany and Europe.

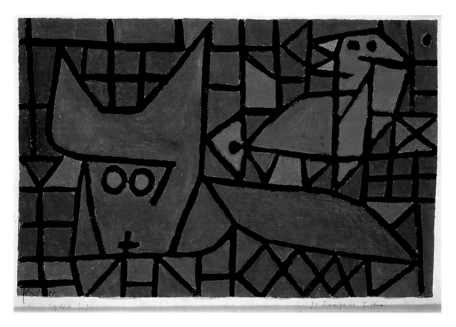

Fig. 14. Paul Klee, Animals in Captivity, 1940, 263, colored paste on paper on cardboard, 31.2 × 48.3 cm. Private collection, Switzerland, with kind permission. ©2010, ProLitteris, Zurich.

Figure 14: Animals in Captivity, 1940

In 'Animals in Captivity' two animals, a fox and a bird, are caught in a cage. They are aware of their hopeless situation. They look at us sadly. The mood is depressed. Klee probably identified himself with these animals in captivity. He felt captive in his 'armored-skin' in his isolation in Berne. In this magnificent painting, we also recognize a peculiarity in the style of Klee's late works: the bordering of areas with thick black lines, the so-called 'beam lines'. This form of representation is often wrongly interpreted as being the result of his thickened and hardened fingers which, it is asserted, would have prevented him from being able to draw fine lines. According to his son's definite testimony, and according to others who knew the artist personally, however, his hands were spared by the illness. The 'beam lines' can thus be interpreted as a simplification, a reduction to the essential that typified his late work, which was characterized by the use of thick outlines.

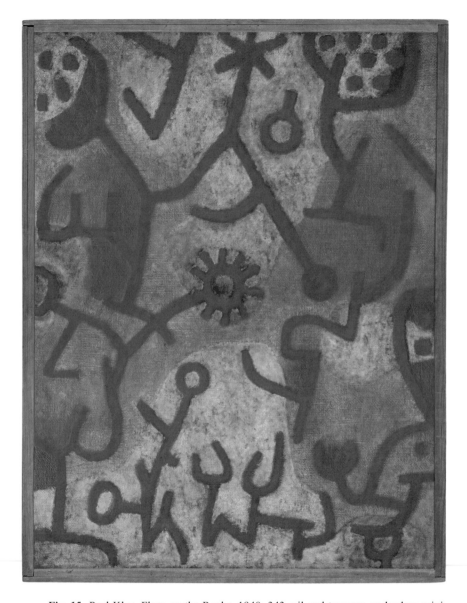

Fig. 15. Paul Klee, Flora on the Rocks, 1940, 343, oil and tempera on burlap; original frame, 90.7 × 70.5 cm. Kunstmuseum Bern, with kind permission. ©2010, ProLitteris, Zurich.

Figure 15: Flora on the Rocks, 1940

The last oil painting entered in Klee's oeuvre catalogue at the end of April 1940, 'Flora on the Rocks', shows a lichen-like floral growth on luminous red- and orange-colored surfaces. Lichens consist of a fungus and an algae that act in symbiosis. The fungus' scaly branches serve the algae as a water and mineral store, while the algae supplies the fungus with organic nutrient. It is only by means of this symbiosis that lichens can survive in marginal environments such as rocks and tree trunks.

Every good partnership involves symbiosis. Paul and Lily Klee enjoyed a harmonious, symbiotic marriage, despite difficult circumstances for both in their last years in Berne. Lily eased her husband's suffering during illness as much as she was able. The picture panel, painted a few months before his death, could be a message from the artist in which he says 'yes' to life, as well as to dying and death. He is ready to bid farewell – conscious of having made good use of his rich gifts during his not so long life; and conscious also that through his creativity he had mastered fate and illness. The last registered oil painting could be a homage to his wife, and at the same time a form of epilogue.

Plants were of great importance to the artist. He collected, dried and pressed them and kept them in glass cases. He knew a great deal about botany. Gardens and parks are important motifs in his creative work. Observing the different stages of nature was intrinsic to him, watching the unfolding, growth and decay made him feel at one with nature and creation. This dialogue with nature not only provided a stimulus for his creativity but also gave him strength during his illness. He hints at this in his now famous statement: 'In the here and now I cannot be understood, for I live as well with the dead as with the unborn. Somewhat nearer the heart of creation than normal – and yet not nearly close enough'.

In May 1940 Paul Klee visited Locarno, in southern Switzerland, for a holiday.

Suddenly his condition worsened and he had to be taken to a private clinic. There, he died on June 29, 1940, in the presence of his wife and his cat Bimbo, which Lily had brought to him from Berne. The death certificate mentions 'myocarditis' as the cause of death. During the simple funeral service at the chapel of the Burgerspital (citizens hospital) in Berne on July 4, 1940, the art historian Georg Schmidt from Basel described Klee as 'the gentlest, most cautious, most delicate, most tender amongst the artists of our time'.

How did the illness of Paul Klee influence his artistic productivity?

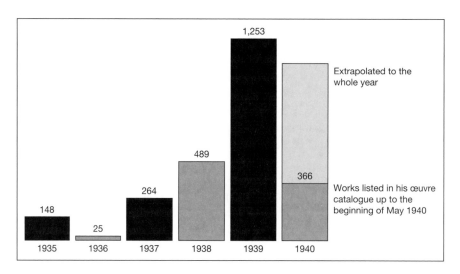

Fig. 16. Artistic production during illness. From Suter H: Paul Klee und seine Krankheit. Berne, Stämpfli, 2006, p 222, with kind permission.

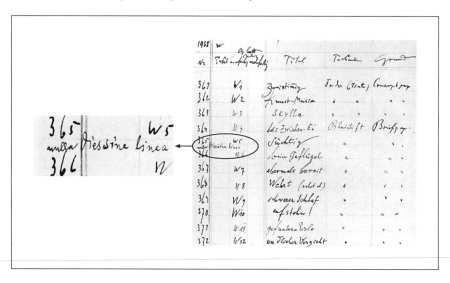

Fig. 17. Page from Klee's oeuvre catalogue of 1938. Zentrum Paul Klee, with kind permission.

Figure 16: Artistic Production during Illness

In 1935 Klee entered 148 works in his oeuvre catalogue, predominantly from the first half of that year. His illness started in summer 1935. It escalated sharply in early 1936, and in that year he was bedridden for a long time and produced only 25 works.

In 1937 there were some periods of improvement. He registered 264 works. In 1938 the number almost doubled. Then the illness worsened. Intuitively, Klee recognized that he probably will not live long. He pulled himself together, and in the face of the inevitable, he was determined to be as productive as possible. In 1939 he increased his output to an almost unbelievable 1,253 works, mainly drawings! In 1940 he still managed 366 works in his last four creative months. Extrapolating from this figure, Klee, had he lived, would have achieved in 1940 a similar annual output to that of 1939 (fig. 16).

Paul Klee's complete oeuvre comprises some 10,000 works. In the 5 years of his illness he produced some 2,500 works – a quarter of his total work. By any measure, it was an outstanding accomplishment!

Figure 17: Page from Klee's Oeuvre Catalogue of 1938

Here is a peculiarity relating to the 366 works of the year 1940. In the oeuvre catalogue of 1938 we find under the number 365 that Klee entered a quotation by the Roman writer Plinius: 'nulla dies sine linea'. This means: 'No day without a line, without a drawing, without creative work'. 1940 was a leap year, having 366 days. Before travelling to the south of Switzerland, surely Klee would have had his scheduled yearly production in mind. With the 366 works of his last 4 creative months, he faithfully adhered to his motto 'nulla dies sine linea'.

Acknowledgements

I would like to thank the following people who were such a pleasure to work with: Prof. Julien Bogousslavsky, MD, and Prof. Michael G. Hennerici, MD, PhD, as main volume editors, Angela Weber, Karger Publishers, as production editor, Robert Haller (Hünibach, Switzerland) as translator, and Dr. Alan George, PhD, London, for reading the English text.

References

Biography
Frey S: Paul Klee, Chronologische Biographie (1933–1941); in: Paul Klee, Das Schaffen im Todesjahr. Berne, Kunstmuseum Bern, 1990, pp 111–132.
Grohmann W: Paul Klee. Geneva, Trois Collines/ Stuttgart, Kohlhammer, 1954, 1965, ed 4, pp 11–96.
Klee F: Paul Klee, Leben und Werk in Dokumenten. Zurich, Diogenes, 1960.
Klee P: Curriculum vitae, Jan 7, 1940. Berne, Zentrum Paul Klee.

Klee P. Briefe an die Familie 1893–1940; Klee F (ed): Cologne, M. Dumont Schauberg, 1979.
Suter H: Paul Klee und seine Krankheit. Berne, Stämpfli, 2006, pp 19–37.

Efforts to Obtain Swiss Citizenship
Suter H: Paul Klee und seine Krankheit. Berne, Stämpfli, 2006, pp 30–31, 266–267.

Illness
Conversations of Hans Suter with Felix Klee, Berne, 1979, 1981, 1983; in Suter H: Paul Klee und seine
 Krankheit. Berne, Stämpfli 2006, p 13.
Frey, S: Paul Klee, Zitate zur Krankengeschichte. Paul Klee's Estate. Berne, Zentrum Paul Klee.
Klee L: Lebenserinnerungen, ab 1942. Paul Klee's Estate. Berne, Zentrum Paul Klee.
Klee P, Klee L: Letters to Will and Gertrud Grohmann, Germany, 1929–1946. Stuttgart, Archiv Will
 Grohmann, Staatsgalerie..
Suter H: Paul Klee und seine Krankheit. Berne, Stämpfli, 2006, pp 39–107.

Paul Klee's Oeuvre Catalogue
Zentrum Paul Klee, Berne.

Illness and Artistic Transfiguration, Interpretations of the Illustrations
Personal interpretations of the author; fully in: Suter H: Paul Klee und seine Krankheit. Berne, Stämpfli,
 2006, pp 16–17, 22–26, 36, 44, 56–57, 66, 84–85, 122–125, 127–239.

Recommended Reading
Giedion-Welcker C: Paul Klee in Selbstzeugnissen und Bilddokumenten. Reinbek/Hamburg, Rowohlt,
 2000.
Glaesemer J: Paul Klee, Handzeichnungen I. Berne, Kunstmuseum Bern, 1973.
Glaesemer J: Paul Klee, Die farbigen Werke im Kunstmuseum Bern. Berne, Kunstmuseum Bern, 1976.
Glaesemer J: Paul Klee, Handzeichnungen III. Berne, Kunstmuseum Bern, 1979.
Glaesemer J: Paul Klee, Handzeichnungen II. Berne, Kunstmuseum Bern, 1984.
Grohmann W: Paul Klee. Geneva, Trois Collines/Stuttgart, Kohlhammer, 1954.
Grohmann W: Der Maler Paul Klee. Cologne, M. DuMont Schauberg, 2003.
Grote L: Erinnerungen an Paul Klee. Munich, Prestel, 1959.
Heim E: Krankheit als Krise und Chance. Stuttgart, Kreuz, 1980.
Hopfengart C: Klee. Vom Sonderfall zum Publikumsliebling. Mainz, Philipp von Zabern, 1989.
Huggler M: Paul Klee, Die Malerei als Blick in den Kosmos. Frauenfeld, Huber, 1969.
Kort P: Paul Klee und die Zeichnungen zur 'nationalsozialistischen Revolution'. Cologne, Walther
 König, 2003.
Klee, Paul, Leben und Werk. Berne, Kunstmuseum Bern/New York, Museum of Modern Art, 1987.
Klee, Paul, Das Schaffen im Todesjahr. Stuttgart, Hatje, 1990.
Klee, Paul, Catalogue raisonné in 9 Bänden. Berne, Benteli, 1998–2004.
Suter H: Paul Klee und seine Krankheit. Berne, Stämpfli, 2006.
Suter H: Paul Klee et sa maladie. Fahrni, 2007.
Suter H: Paul Klee and His Illness. Basel, Karger, 2010.

Dr. med. Dr. h.c Hans Suter
Spezialarzt für Dermatologie und Venerologie FMH
Lueg
CH–3617 Fahrni (Switzerland)
Tel. +41 33 437 59 51, Fax +41 33 437 59 52, E-Mail info@sammlung-suter.ch

Bogousslavsky J, Hennerici MG, Bäzner H, Bassetti C (eds): Neurological Disorders in Famous Artists – Part 3. Front Neurol Neurosci. Basel, Karger, 2010, vol 27, pp 29–45

....

The Last Myth of Giorgio de Chirico: Neurological Art

Julien Bogousslavsky

Center for Brain and Nervous System Disorders, and Neurorehabilitation Services, Genolier Swiss Medical Network, Clinique Valmont, Montreux, Switzerland

Abstract

Giorgio de Chirico is one of the most admired and at the same time most discredited painters of the 20th century. As the 'inventor' of metaphysical painting, he has been considered as a precursor of Surrealism, while his later works have been harshly criticized as representative of the painter's decay. The mystery and dream-like atmosphere irradiating from his works has led to speculations that de Chirico may have taken his inspiration from migraine attacks or complex partial seizures. However, a careful study of his life and his own writings suggests that while de Chirico probably suffered from recurrent malaria, he had neither migraines nor epilepsy. De Chirico also denied that dreams were a major source of his inspiration, but he insisted on his fertile inner imagery, which allowed him to put in a new, poetic, often conflictual perspective, places and objects, which he had actually *seen* (Hofgarten arcades, Italian piazzas, statues, antique ruins, etc.) in Athens, Munich, Florence, Turin, Ferrare, and other towns. De Chirico was accused of self-plagiarism because he commonly used his former themes in new works, sometimes in what may look like servile copies of his early paintings. This 'replay syndrome' is quite unique in modern art, which has been dominated by the obligation, dogma and cult of newness and renewal. At odds with most of his contemporaries, Andy Warhol suggested that de Chirico made such recurrent series because 'he liked it'. Indeed, as a lifelong admirer of Nietzsche, de Chirico may just have applied the philosopher's concept of the 'eternal return', in which one is supposed to live and accomplish tasks that one would want to repeat forever. In that way, de Chirico's work should not be considered as that of a genius who fell into decadence, but may appear as a continuous, organized process to which organic brain dysfunction never contributed.

Copyright © 2010 S. Karger AG, Basel

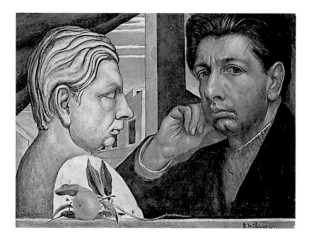

Fig. 1. Giorgio de Chirico. Autoportrait (1922). Courtesy Fondazione de Chirico, Rome. ©2010, ProLitteris, Zurich.

'Wind, wind that cools my burning cheeks. And the terrible battle began. Broken heads fell, and skulls shone as if they were ivory'
Giorgio de Chirico
The Statue's Desire, 1912

This volume is the third of a series focusing on the occurrence of neurological disorders in famous artists and how their creativity and production was subsequently modified. The Italian painter Giorgio de Chirico (fig. 1), 'the most astonishing of modern painters' according to Guillaume Apollinaire in 1913 [Taylor, 2002, p. 16], is regularly quoted as such, since he may have suffered from migraine or epilepsy, which supposedly greatly influenced his artistic output, starting with his 'metaphysical period', and during most of his life [Blanke and Landis, 2003; Podoll et al., 2001]. Migraine in particular is a great classic here, and a book on de Chirico entitled 'Arte emicranica' has even been devoted to the topic [Podoll and Nicola,, 2003]. To most observers, de Chirico's paintings radiate a particular strangeness, which is certainly at the origin of the speculations on specific brain conditions which may have predisposed the painter's style. However, when discussing medical issues in his Mémoires, de Chirico [1965] insisted on episodes of intestinal pains and fever, while any potential neurological dysfunction is scarcely mentioned: only two episodes of nonspecific headache and one episode compatible with complex visual hallucinations are cited, with no report at all of the basic visual changes associated with migraine aura or any alteration of consciousness. While fighting each other [Blanke and Landis,

2004; Podoll and Nicola, 2004], migraine and epilepsy enthusiasts have focused on other writings of de Chirico, including poetic essays such as 'Monsieur Dudron' or 'Hebdomeros'. Indeed, these texts report a wide panorama of visual, sensory, and internal phenomena presented in an oneiric and imaginative style, which has even allowed a literary comparison with 'Les Chants de Maldoror' by Lautréamont, published a few decades earlier, and which would become one of the fetish books of the Surrealists. It is of course not impossible that certain of these phenomena were experienced by the painter himself, although this seems rather unlikely as he never mentioned them in his autobiographical writings (one may argue that 'any' writing is somewhat autobiographical, but this is another matter). But it must be acknowledged that there is no recognized fact or clue in de Chirico's life and memories that hallucinations played any role in his inspiration. Moreover, it may be particularly reductionist to underline a direct link between an unproven and unlikely neurological condition, and the genesis of the work of one of the most important painters of the 20th century, as if migrainous or epileptic hallucinations simply could explain the 'Enigma' or 'Ariadne' series, or the 'Bagni misteriosi'. It is also reductionist, by the way, to try to explain the source of the 'metaphysical paintings' by specific dreams, a claim which has been advanced by the Surrealists, but was clearly denied by de Chirico himself, who stated several times that his inspiration did not come from his dreams [Baldacci, 1998, p. 409]. Several myths have grown around de Chirico as a man and as an artist. 'Neuro-artistic' hypotheses on migraine, epilepsy, dreamy states, etc., appear to have built up a new de Chirico myth: neurological art, which it is now time to destroy.

Short Biography of Giorgio de Chirico

De Chirico was born in Volos, Greece, in 1888, 3 years before his brother Alberto, who was also to become famous in arts under the pseudonym of Alberto Savinio. After staying for some time in Athens, the de Chirico brothers went to Munich, where Giorgio studied at the Akademie der Bildenden Kunst, being influenced by Boecklin's and Klinger's paintings. In 1909, on his way to Milan, where he would discover the writings of Nietzsche ('the most profound of all poets'), de Chirico stopped in Florence, where his memory of the piazza Santa Croce would give him the inspiration for what is considered his first metaphysical painting ('The Enigma of an Autumn Afternoon'). After staying in Florence in 1910, he went to Paris in 1911, stopping for one and a half days in Turin, where he was greatly struck by the architecture of piazzas. A second trip to Turin took place in 1912, where he rediscovered the piazzas, as well as statues, which would inspire him for the statues of the 'political man' in his paintings. 1912 was also the year of the Ariadne series. In 1914, the young art dealer Paul Guillaume offered de Chirico a contract, in which he would pay 120 francs against 6 works per month. New trips to Turin, Florence, and finally Ferrare, occurred in 1915, where de Chirico had to complete his military duties (he was considered a draft dodger and a deserter in 1911–1912). In 1916, de Chirico met Tristan Tzara in Zurich, who was just initiating the Dada movement, and discovered the writings of Otto Weininger who with Nietzsche and Schopenhauer formed a philosophical triad. Along with the futurist painter Carlo Carrá, de Chirico was sent to the Military Reserve Hospital in Villa del Seminario, just outside Ferrare in 1917. This was a convalescent hospital used mainly for soldiers with nervous instability. This was apparently not the case for de Chirico who was sent there upon recommendation from his friend, the painter Filippo de Pisis [Baldacci, 1998]. According to what the Surrealists would later comment upon, the metaphysical period of de Chirico's work ends in 1917–1918, while he first used the term 'classical painting' to describe his own work in 1919. From that time on, the pictorial evolution of de Chirico has been controversial in the art world, and his changes of style have often been qualified as 'degenerescence', while his habit of 'copying' previous works from the metaphysical period sometimes antedating them ('authentic fakes'), has also been considered a sign of artistic degradation. However, in parallel, many new topics appeared in de Chirico's work, including dummies, antique figures inhabited by temples and ruins, gladiators, the 'bagni misteriosi' series, etc., together with classical-looking portraits, still lives, and landscapes, about which de Chirico emphasized his rediscovery of ancient Renaissance tempera and oil techniques. This artistic controversy was exacerbated in 1925–1930 during a new stay in Paris, when violent opposition developed with previous friends from the surrealist movement (mainly André Breton and Paul Éluard), who publically stated that only his metaphysical works were of value, and energetically criticized the exhibition of his recent paintings organized by his new dealer Léonce Rosenberg. De Chirico subsequently stayed in Milan, New York, and after the war, Rome. In 1974, he was elected to the seat of Jacques Lipschitz at the Académie des Beaux-Arts in Paris, where he stated in his reception speech: 'I wish to add that I never belonged to any artistic movement and that my principal concern has always been to paint well'. Two years later he had his first heart attack; a second one in 1978, at age 90, caused his death 6 weeks later.

De Chirico's 'Migraine'

Migraine has frequently been emphasized as a potential source of inspiration of certain artists and writers [Fuller and Gale, 1988; see Vicks and

Table 1. Arguments for and against migraine

Habit of not leaving home without a metal box with almost six pills against headache	Only reported in 'Monsieur Dudron'
Positive family history of headaches [father, brother(?)]	Nonspecific for migraine. Other diseases in the family, in particular malaria
Headaches	Reported only twice in the Mémoires 1965, pp 48–49, 56], with no migrainous characteristics
Abdominal discomfort	Absence of reported nausea or vomiting
Positive effect of sleep	A positive effect was reported on abdominal pain and fever
Avoidance of eggs	De Chirico only mentioned that he knew that eggs should be avoided when taking sulfamides for fever [de Chirico, 1965, pp 209–210)
Elementary visual hallucinations/geometric scotomas	Not mentioned in the Mémoires, but in 'Hebdomeros' [p 105]

Sexton-Radek, 2005, for a thorough review], including Lewis Caroll (Alice in Wonderland syndrome), William Blake, and even the unlikely Picasso. While de Chirico hardly ever mentioned experiencing headaches, migraine remains the most often quoted of his potential 'neurological diseases'. It is possible that André Breton was initially responsible for this suggestion, when he claimed that Apollinaire had told him that de Chirico mentioned that he had 'cenesthetic' phenomena.

Several years after the painter's death, a group of authors emphasized the 'migraine hypothesis' as a significant source of de Chirico's art [Podoll and Robinson, 2000; Podoll et al., 2001; Podoll and Nicola, 2003]. While these authors recognized that headache had never been a significant complaint of de Chirico, they hypothesized that de Chirico suffered from the uncommon 'migraine sine migraine' form, and listed a whole series of tentatively migrainous phenomena, which could have affected him: nausea, photophobia, abdominal discomfort, gustatory hallucinations, scotomas and more complex visual hallucinations, autoscopia, recurrent dreams, feeling of depersonalization-derealization, déjà-vu/jamais-vu, and macrosomatognosia. The first problem here is that without a suggestive association, these phenomena taken in isolation bear absolutely no specificity for migraine or any other neurological disease. Secondly, nearly all these phenomena are completely absent from de Chirico's Mémoires [1965]. Certain passages in other writings, mainly 'Hebdomeros' and

'Une Aventure de Monsieur Dudron' were interpreted as clues for de Chirico's migraine, because the above-mentioned phenomena can be identified in the text. However, it is a rather risky shortcut to imply that the feelings experienced by fictional figures in an author's writings correspond to experiences of that particular author (even if de Chirico once said 'Hebdomeros, this is me!'), especially when they are absent from autobiographical writings. Table 1 shows the main clues for migraine, and the corresponding counter-arguments.

If the work of de Chirico is examined, it is difficult to find convincing depictions of migrainous visual phenomena. The example which seems the most compatible is the representation of water in the 'Bagni misteriosi' series (fig. 2), but it bears no specificity. The lithograph illustrations for Apollinaire's 'Calligrammes', published in 1930 by Gallimard, have often been quoted as another example [Podoll and Nicola, 2003]. However, de Chirico himself explained his inspiration quite differently to the Belgian collector René Gaffé, to whom he had sold his personal copy of the book enriched with original drawings and watercolor adjunctions [Bogousslavsky, 2003, 2005b]: 'For the lithographs under your eyes, he told me, I took inspiration from the memories of the years 1913–1914: I had just met the poet. I was reading with avidity his verses in which suns and stars are frequently mentioned. At the same time, by a mental phenomenon, which is familiar to me and which is often reflected in my paintings, I was thinking of Italy, its towns and its mines. Suddenly, for me, through a lightning which makes you discover beside you the object you are thinking of, these suns and stars were coming back on earth like peaceful emigrants. They were probably off in the sky, since I was seeing them being switched on at the door of many houses. Was it unreasonable to establish on the fountain of my mind and on the state of my visions the lithographs which would coexist with the poetic scales played by Apollinaire as a true visionary?' [Gaffé, 1946]. This quotation, by the way, is of utmost importance in understanding the creative process of de Chirico, since it underscores his inner visualization of specific items during the uprising of imaginative thinking, with no suggestion at all for 'hallucinations', either elementary or complex.

De Chirico's 'Epilepsy'

The idea that de Chirico may have experienced partial complex seizures is more recent than the migraine hypothesis, and in fact, it seems to have developed as a reaction against the latter, which was thought to be unlikely [Blanke and Landis, 2003]. Indeed, the subjects and items appearing in de Chirico's work are closer to oneiric depictions reported in certain temporal lobe seizures than to the geometrical deformations and blurring of migrainous auras

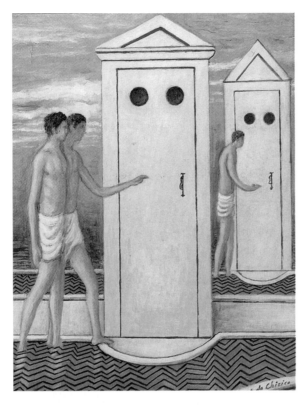

Fig. 2. Bagni misteriosi: Les Cabines Mystérieuses (1935). Courtesy Fondazione de Chirico, Rome. ©2010, ProLitteris, Zurich.

[Bogousslavsky, 2003]. However, it is not because oneiric items appear in a canvas that it means that the painter had hallucinations or seizures. Moreover, many of de Chirico's works represent complex, highly symbolic, constructs (pictures into pictures, temples and ruins inside people), which suggest a well-structured, sophisticated mental activity, rather than the production of the twilight or confusional state seen in partial complex seizures. Olfactory-gustatory hallucinations have also been emphasized as a sign in favor of temporal epilepsy in de Chirico [Blanke and Landis, 2003]. However, these so-called hallucinations were reported in his Mémoires by the painter himself as a special sensitivity to odors, but without features of hallucinations or even as a trigger to other experiences or neurological phenomena. Ten olfactory-gustatory experiences can be delineated in the Mémoires, and they do not suggest a pathological phenomenon (table 2).

Table 2. Reported olfactory-gustatory experiences in Mémoires

Bad breath of his teacher Barbieri	p 29
Marvelous taste of grapes	p 49
Taste of phenic acid	p 69
Musty smell in Vallombroso	p 70
Foul smell in army buildings in Florence	p 86
Foul smell in army buildings in Ferrara	p 90
Phenic acid smell in a lady's building	p 90
Taste of a fruit juice (tamarind)	p 95
Marvelous taste of roasted lamb	p 130
Strange odors upon arrival in New York	p 157

Table 3. Arguments for and against partial complex seizures

Motion sickness	Totally nonspecific
Abdominal pains	Totally nonspecific, other medical reasons present
Short duration of pain is more suggestive of epilepsy than migraine	Episodes lasting several days also reported
Olfactory-gustatory 'hallucinations'	Hallucinatory nature unlikely (table 2)
Visual 'hallucinations'	Only one suggestive episode (disappearance of Longhi into the pavement [de Chirico, 1965, p 110])
Interictal personality traits (sensation of personal destiny, paranoia, philosophical preoccupation, preservative themes in painting)	Totally nonspecific
'Malaises'	No loss or alteration of consciousness, only one report of fearing to faint and fall [de Chirico, 1965, pp 68–70]
Jamais-vu	Once(?) (Santa Croce, 1910), nonspecific
Autoscopy	Speculation based on some autoportraits of the painter with two different representations of himself (fig. 1), but an autoscopic phenomenon was never reported

The potential arguments in favor of partial complex seizures have been summarized by Blanke and Landis [2003]. They appear in table 3 together with a critical appreciation.

A last phenomenon which has been interpreted as a sign of possible brain dysfunction is the occurrence of a premonitory feeling on three occasions: his father's death (after seeing a black sheet at a balcony) [p 51]; his mother's death (dream) [p 162], and his visit to the painter Laprade (dream in which he had seen the canvas on which Laprade was working when he arrived in his studio the next day) [p 74]. However, such phenomena are not uncommon in a lifetime, and no associated manifestation suggests that they were related to an epileptic phenomenon in the case of de Chirico. Overall, the possibility that de Chirico had epileptic seizures seems as speculative and unlikely as the role of migraine in his artistic production.

However, aside from the epilepsy speculations, it is absolutely correct that 'vision' always was a critical issue in de Chirico's life and work, as underscored by himself: 'I try to express as strongly as possible the images and fantasies which haunt my mind' [De Chirico Catalogue, 2009]. The vocabulary of vision has indeed always been used and emphasized about de Chirico, as exemplified by his dealer Paul Guillaume in a conference at the Vieux-Colombier in November 1918: 'De Chirico paints only when a sudden and fatal vision appears in his mind' [De Chirico Catalogue, 2009]. This suggests a developed, active, imagination, and in the Mémoires, several paragraphs show instances of this peculiar power of inner visualization: 'The image of a fat gentleman with a red face, sitting at a table, a napkin knotted around his neck, who, armed with a fork and knife, prepares himself to attack an enormous Florentine-style steak placed in his plate' [p 209]. The famous story of the genesis of the 'first' metaphysical painting is another vivid example: 'Let me recount how I had the revelation of a picture that I will show this year at the Salon d'Automne, entitled Enigma of an Autumn Afternoon. One clear autumnal afternoon I was sitting on a bench in the middle of the Piazza Santa Croce in Florence. It was of course not the first time I had seen this square. I had just come out of a long and painful intestinal illness, and I was in a nearly morbid state of sensitivity. The whole world, down to the marble of the buildings and the fountains, seemed to me to be convalescent. In the middle of the square rises a statue of Dante draped in a long cloak, holding his works clasped against his body, his laurel-crowned head bent thoughtfully earthward. The statue is in white marble, but time has given it a grey cast, very agreeable to the eye. The autumn sun, warm and unloving, lit the statue and the church façade. Then I had the strange impression that I was looking at these things for the first time, and the composition of my picture came to my mind's eye. Now each time I look at this painting I again see that moment. Nevertheless the moment is an enigma to me for it is inexplicable.

And I like also to call the work which sprang from it an enigma' [Soby, 1955, p 251]. This extraordinary, precise, description demonstrates this critical interaction between de Chirico's imaginary inner vision and his creative process, and by the way it also gives an interesting light on why the painter called so many of his early metaphysical paintings 'enigmas'.

Medical Issues and Diseases Reported by de Chirico

In his Mémoires, de Chirico precisely reported the medical problems which he developed during in his life. Usually details abound, and for that reason it is very unlikely that he failed to report any disorder (such as migrainous or epileptic episodes) which might have altered or modified his own work. The most common problem quoted by de Chirico refers to attacks of fever with abdominal pain and general weakness, which can most likely be explained by malaria which de Chirico himself acknowledged to have caught in Greece [p 35], and which his father and other family members also had. These attacks are discussed at least eight times in the Mémoires [1965, pp 14, 35, 48–49, 53, 68–70, 72–73, 98–100, 207–211], only once with a headache [pp 48–49], and never with any focal neurological dysfunction. These episodes lasted up to two weeks, resolving spontaneously or with hot towels, rest and laudanum. De Chirico attributed these episodes either to malaria [p 35] or to rheumatic fevers [pp 207–211]. Other medical conditions include cranial trauma as a child, without loss of consciousness [p 21], elbow pain [p 26], painful twisted neck [p 56], melancholia [pp 68–70], and sea sickness [p 156]. While de Chirico reported that he was nearly excluded from being drafted because of an 'oblique chin' [pp 86–87], he spent several months in the army during World War I, without known medical problems, except the fever-pain attacks. In 1917, because of 'fragile health' [De Chirico Catalogue, 2009], but in fact mainly because he was supported and recommended by Filippo de Pisis [Baldacci, 1998], de Chirico was sent for duty at the Military Reserve Hospital of Villa del Seminario. Soldiers with nervous disorders were sent there for convalescence, but this was not the case of de Chirico who was assigned to the place as military personnel, being allowed to use his free time to paint. Overall, we know little about de Chirico's doctors, as he mentioned only one medical consultation, with a 'celebrity' (Professor Grocco), who saw him in 1910 in Florence for one of the abdominal attacks, but only prescribed rest [pp 68–70]. In conclusion, after examining the above-mentioned medical issues reported by de Chirico in his Mémoires, it is indeed difficult to find any suggestive clue for an underlying, chronic or intermittent, neurological illness of any sort.

Surrealism, Dreams, and the Issue of Change of Style

While the Surrealists bear the main responsibility for the claim that de Chirico's metaphysical paintings relate to dreams and dreaming, the initial suggestion came much earlier, as shown by the quotation from Ardengo Soffici by Apollinaire in his 'Chroniques d'art' article of July 14, 1914: 'His work resembles no other, either antique or modern (…) one may define it as a dream writing'.

The Surrealists emphasized the mysterious poetry of de Chirico as an expression of the unconscious which manifested itself during dreams, but both de Chirico and Savinio always claimed that dreams were never at the origin of their creative inspiration [Baldacci, 1998]. André Breton was fascinated by a 'veritable modern mythology' [Breton, 1920] which he had discovered in the 'Child's Brain', the first de Chirico painting that he had bought in 1919, and the apparent disconnection between the titles and the subjects of the paintings was interpreted as a typical surrealist 'automatism'. Indeed, this was subsequently heavily used or copied by Max Ernst and René Magritte, along with other surrealist painters. While de Chirico denied the influence of dreams on his work, he may not have been completely honest on that matter, since his violent disputes with his former surrealist friends ('the champions among champions of modernist imbecility' [de Chirico Mémoires, 1965, p 77], which arose after 1925, obviously influenced his statements. Indeed, the role of sleep and dreams is already suggested by de Chirico's sleeping Ariadne series of 1912–1913. Later, he even wrote 'Dreams' for 'La Révolution Surréaliste' in 1924, and the oneiric tuning of 'Hebdomeros', published in 1929, is obvious. But when the Surrealists felt that the unconscious poetry of dreams had left de Chirico's works, after 1918 (especially after 1924), they condemned him and his paintings without appeal [Breton, 1928]. While we may accept that dreaming was perhaps not a major source of de Chirico's inspiration, for the observer his work is a strong stimulus to 'awake dreams', and the 2009 de Chirico retrospective exhibition in Paris was entitled 'The fabric of dreams' [De Chirico Catalogue, 2009].

De Chirico never gave an 'explanation' for his 'change of style' in the 1920s when he was accused by the Surrealists of deception and treason of his metaphysical work, but in his Mémoires [1965, pp 206, 227], he affirmed that contrary to the legend, he had never left or rejected his metaphysical paintings period. The issue was very hot, because Breton and his friends had used de Chirico's work to support a large part of the ideas which underlie surrealism, and Max Ernst recalled that in the 1930s, when he visited de Chirico in his studio, together with Breton and Giacometti [Taylor, 2002, pp. 171–175], 'he showed us a series of paintings which had been done in the lowest postcard style. All of them were of Venice, Italy. After we had seen 10 or 12 paintings suddenly André Breton became furious and insulted Chirico in the most horrible manner. Chirico did not mind at all. He said "Oh, if you do not like Venice I can show you some views of Naples". And so he showed us some views of Naples in the same postcard style (…) André spoke to Chirico about his former work and Chirico pretended it was nothing at all, less than s***. Chirico said "It is the easiest thing in the world to make this kind of painting even right now if some stupid people could be found to buy them".' In his interpretation, Max Ernst compared de Chirico to Rimbaud or Duchamp in some kind of 'self-destruction' attempt, and stated that in fact he admired the way the painter went to the very end of that intention.

At the end of his metaphysical painting period, around 1919–1920, de Chirico declared himself a 'classical painter', but several of his earlier works, such as the portrait of his brother Alberto in Renaissance clothes and surroundings, also share this 'classical' flavor. De Chirico defined himself as the 'rediscoverer of great painting, buried and forgotten by the whole world' [De Chirico, 1965, p 103]. Indeed, classicism is perhaps the strongest link between de Chirico's different periods, and when one looks at his 70-year production, it remains striking how strong the overlap is between the observed changes and an obvious continuity of the classicism of his style(s), which contributes to the uniqueness of his work and gives it its peculiar mystery. De Chirico repeatedly stated that nobody really understood his work: 'nobody ever understood anything of it, either at the time, or nowadays' [De Chirico, 1965, p 77]. He put his statements in the perspective of a general artistic decadence, which corresponded to a 'rampant narcissism' of artists in what he called the 'comedy of modern art' [Taylor, 2002, p 17].

In the discussion on de Chirico's work, the term 'metaphysical painting' also seems to have covered different meanings over the time. Breton already wanted to replace the term 'metaphysical' by 'metapsychological'. In de Chirico's own vocabulary, the term was used for the 'discovery of a new world' [Rubin et al., 1983, p 249]. While de Chirico's metaphysical paintings always represent well-defined objects, they also underline an absence of logic of their inner world, and certain mythical characteristics where each sign may have several faces. De Chirico stated: 'This is the absurd and quiet beauty of matter itself, which is "metaphysical" for me, as are metaphysical these objects with such a frankness of colors and precision of shapes that they can be placed at the antipodes of any confusion and any nebulosity' [Baldacci, 1998, p 409]. It is critical to realize that de Chirico's metaphysical paintings thus bear nothing obscure, depicting what is actually real and visible, but also something beyond what is just apparent. Indeed, de Chirico often represents worlds, which are 'appearances', such as theater sets, houses without function, empty-looking squares, or objects with no support to maintain them. Animals, such as horses, typically look immobile, like statues, although they are depicted in full stride. Human beings initially appeared as minuscule figures, before being transformed into statues, dummies, antique figures inhabited by temples and ruins, and impersonal figures only identified through their tools and functions (gladiators, warriors). Gordon Onslow Ford described this world as 'de Chirico City': an instantly recognizable world of statues, clocks, trains, smokestacks situated within an eerily silent urban square with arcades and empty spaces, with an atmosphere of premonition, solitude, ecstasy and immobility [Taylor, 2002, p 15]. The fascinating result is still reinforced by an 'initiatic' aspect of the works, with a subsequent feeling of gratification to the observer for having been able to penetrate into that strange world.

As I emphasized before, de Chirico's world is that of 'vision', his vision which is typically contagious to the observer. Indeed, de Chirico always painted objects which he had actually seen (such as the statue of Giovanni Battista Bottero in Turin, the Italian piazzas, factories, or the arcades of the Hofgarten in Munich). In that way, de Chirico simply represented on the canvas what his actual vision had registered, and never the fruit of pure imagination or any presumed 'hallucination'. Imagination only subsequently intervened for the ensemble presentation and structuration of all these items just extracted from the real. Seen through that perspective, de Chirico's 'changes of style' may only have a minor importance as a reflect of his own evolution, and probably less than those changes observed in other painters, without (Picasso, Kandinsky, Picabia) or with a brain lesion (de Kooning, Corinth, Reuterswärd, Gernez) [Bogousslavsky and Hennerici, 2007]. As often, Marcel Duchamp may have made the most clever remark at the time, in 1943: 'His admirers could not follow him and they decided that the Chirico second manner had lost its original flame. But posterity will perhaps have a word to say' [Rubin et al., 1983, p 274].

De Chirico's 'Ambiguity'

'Ambiguity', i.e. an open door to multiple interpretations and imaginary completions, is a critical feature of the artistic value of a painting, as emphasized by Zeki [1999]. A self-obvious example is unfinished works which allow further mental elaboration into several 'solutions' by the observer. 'Ambiguity' can also arise from certain conflicts between specific aspects of a work of art, such as its topic, pictorial matter, colors, etc. In de Chirico's work, 'ambiguity' is indeed prominent at several levels, which may explain a part of the mystery and fascination that it exerts on the observer.

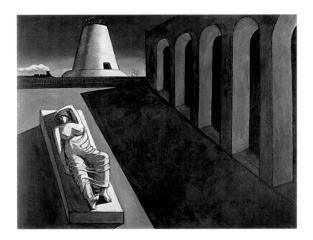

Fig. 3. La Statue Silencieuse (1913). The painter emphasized the gross shapes of the statue of Ariadne, in particular the arm surrounding the head, and the breasts. Courtesy Fondazione de Chirico, Rome. ©2010, ProLitteris, Zurich.

The high quality of the pictorial oil or tempera material is often in apparent contradiction with rather gross shapes of certain items and figures, such as trains (which look more like toys), or 'poorly-drawn' faces or limbs of subjects (Ariadne's arm or chest in some works of the Ariadne series; fig. 3), or over-simplified buildings and arcades. De Chirico's 'white light' [Rubin et al., 1983] usually contrasts with brightly colored objects and does not undergo expected modulations in the different parts of the work, similarly to Henry Rousseau's paintings. The apparently very geometrical perspective of piazzas often leads to a switch from a 3-dimensional to a 2-dimensional representation, which reminds the observer that a painting indeed is a flat object; in spite of the often well-marked shadows (sometimes contrasting with absent, though expected, other shadows), this phenomenon contradicts the sacrosanct illusion of depth, being completely at odds with the common rules of landscape representation. Moreover, different parts of the same work often do not follow the same rules of perspective, leading to a particularly strong visual impression (fig. 4). Contrary to the geometrical system used in cubism, which 'deconstructs' well-identified objects into small non-figurative elements, de Chirico's geometrical structures typically correspond to assemblages of recognizable objects (rulers, set squares) reconstructed into new, unknown, frames and scaffoldings.

De Chirico is certainly one of the 20th century painters who have stimulated some of the most intense controversies [Rubin et al., 1983], and the 'ambi-

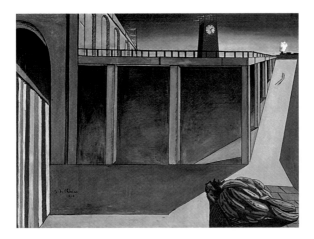

Fig. 4. La Gare Montparnasse (1914). A visual conflict is produced by the schematic perspective of the buildings, while the street on the right does not follow the rules of perspective, leading to a three- to two-dimensional switch. Courtesy Fondazione de Chirico, Rome. ©2010, ProLitteris, Zurich.

guity' which can be identified at several levels in his work is no stranger to such disagreements. The recurrence of themes (statues, Ariadne, trains, walls, arcades, piazzas, etc.), which is in contrast with the unexpected appearance of unusual pictorial objects (artichokes, bananas …) certainly also contributes to a feeling of ambiguity which has expressed itself over the years in extreme judgments oscillating between supreme philosophical depth and grotesque provocation, and which has led certain authors to emphasize a potential neurological dysfunction at the origin of de Chirico's work.

We do not know the brain mechanisms which underlie creativity, in particular extraordinary creativity, such as in art geniuses. The middle frontal gyrus appears to be involved in interpreting certain conflicting aspects which can be found in art works (for instance Fauve paintings with unusual colors for usual objects and buildings) [Zeki, 1999]. A loosening of associations has also been emphasized, but contrary to what may be associated with schizophrenia, a self-organization may then take place and lead to creative works [Andreasen, 2005]. In that way, creativity may start by a disorganizing process, making links between remembered forms and structures which have not been previously linked together, and leading to 'newness'. While the brain regions active during randomly wandering free associations involve the frontal-parietal-temporal association cortex, it is very likely that the processes of creativity involve a more global brain activity ('the whole brain') [Bogousslavsky, 2005a].

De Chirico's Replay Syndrome

De Chirico is well known for his series of painting themes (Ariadne, piazzas, interiors, gladiators, archeologists, bagni misteriosi, etc.). But what is somewhat unique is his propensity to go back to themes apparently abandoned years before, sometimes in what can appear as servile copies of original works dating back to several decades earlier. Since he even antedated some of these new works, de Chirico was not only accused of self-plagiarism, but also of making fake de Chiricos! A famous example is the realization of no less than 18 new versions (most of them being nearly identical copies) of 'The Disquieting Muses' between the original of 1918 and 1962. This replay syndrome has usually been strongly criticized, and used as an example reflecting the decadence of the painter and his loss of creativity [De Chirico Catalogue, 2009]. Following this interpretation, these 'repeated repetitions' would have corresponded to a disappearance of new inner imagery, with a barrening of inspiration renewal [Bogousslavsky, 2003]. Along with the ambient criticism of de Chirico's new works after his metaphysical period, and with the active support of the Surrealists, this is indeed the interpretation which has largely prevailed to date [Pierrard, 2009]. A 'viscosity' of personality, which has been reported in epileptics, has also been advanced by proponents of partial complex seizures in de Chirico [Blanke and Landis, 2003, 2004]. However, a few other tracks probably need to be better explored on the issue of de Chirico's replay syndrome, especially within the frame of the complex personality of this artist. In a 1982 interview, Andy Warhol expressed another opinion which may lead to completely different interpretations: 'De Chirico repeated the same images throughout his life. I believe he did it not only because people and dealers asked him to do it. But because he liked it and viewed repetition as a way of expressing himself' [Taylor, 2002, p 164]. Warhol also acknowledged that de Chirico had markedly influenced him for the realization of his own repetitive series (Marilyn, Mao, Campbell Soup, etc.). The hypothesis that de Chirico actually deeply *enjoyed* repeating subjects and paintings is convincing, and it is in agreement with the influence of Nietzsche on him that de Chirico always recognized. In the introduction to De Chirico's Mémoires, Pierre Mazars wrote: 'I asked de Chirico one day what had inspired the light and atmosphere in his metaphysical paintings. – This is Nietzsche! He answered. Particularly the reading of Ecce Homo'. One has to remember that what Nietzsche proposed as replacement to the Christian concept of salute is what he called the 'eternal return', which is to look for and accomplish tasks that one would want to repeat forever. 'Live in the way that you would like to live again' summarized Nietzsche in one of his famous aphorisms. It is possible that Giorgio de Chirico just applied the formula to himself and his work, leaving it to us to decrypt one of his most profound and intriguing enigmas.

References

Andreasen NC: The Creating Brain. The Neuroscience of Genius. New York, Dana Press, 2005
Apollinaire G: Nouveaux peintres. Paris Journal, July 14, 1914.
Baldacci P: Chirico. La métaphysique, 1888–1919. Paris, Flammarion, 1998.
Blanke O, Landis T: The metaphysical art of Giorgio de Chirico. Migraine or epilepsy? Eur Neurol 2003; 50:191–194.
Blanke O, Landis T: Giorgio de Chirico: intricate links between spiritual fevers, metaphysical art, and the interictal temporal lobe syndrome. Eur Neurol 2004;51:186–187.
Bogousslavsky J: The neurology of art – the example of Giorgio de Chirico. Eur Neurol 2003;50:89–190.
Bogousslavsky J: Artistic creativity, style and brain disorders. Eur Neurol 2005a;54:103–111.
Bogousslavsky J: De Parallèlement à Chanson Complète. Peintres, poètes et livres, un âge d'or, 1900–1939. Plagneise-Maneise, Amitiés France-Helvétie, 2005b.
Bogousslavsky J, Hennerici MG (eds): Neurological Disorders in Famous Artists – Part 2. Front Neurol Neurosci. Basel, Karger, 2007, vol. 22.
Breton A: in Littérature. Paris, 1920.
Breton A: Le surréalisme et la peinture. Paris, NRF, 1928.
De Chirico G: Une aventure de M. Dudron. Paris, L'âge d'or, 1945.
De Chirico G: Mémoires. Préface de Pierre Mazars. Paris, La table ronde, 1965.
De Chirico G: Hebdomeros. Collection L'âge d'or. Paris, Flammarion, 1983.
De Chirico Catalogue: Giorgio de Chirico, la fabrique des rêves. Paris, Musée d'Art Moderne de la Ville de Paris, Paris musées, 2009.
Fuller GN, Gale MV: Migraine aura as artistic inspiration. BMJ 1988;297:1670–1672.
Gaffé R: Giorgio de Chirico le voyant. Bruxelles, Private edition, 1946.
Pierrard J: Le chaos Chirico. La trajectoire chahutée d'un maître du moderne. Le Point Feb. 19, 2009, p 86.
Podoll K, Nicola U: L'aura di Giorgio de Chirico. Arte emicranica e pittura metafisica. Milan, Mimesis, 2003.
Podoll K, Nicola U: The illness of Giorgio de Chirico – Migraine or epilepsy? Eur Neurol 2004;51:186.
Podoll K, Robinson D: Migraine experience as artistic inspiration in a contemporary artist. J R Soc Med 2000;93:263–265.
Podoll K, Robinson D, Nicola U: The migraine of Giorgio de Chirico. 1. History of illness. Neurol Psychiat Brain Res 2001;9:139–156.
Rubin W, Schmied W, Clair J: Giorgio De Chirico. Paris, Centre Georges Pompidou, Musée National d'Art Moderne, 1983.
Soby JT: Giorgio de Chirico. New York, Museum of Modern Art, 1955.
Taylor M (ed): Giorgio de Chirico and the myth of Ariadne. Philadelphia, Philadelphia Museum of Art, 2002.
Vick RM, Sexton-Radek K: Art and migraine: researching the relationship between artmaking and pain experience. Art Ther 2005;22:193–294.
Zeki S: Inner Vision. An Exploration of Art and the Brain. Oxford, Oxford University Press, 1999.

Julien Bogousslavsky, MD
Center for Brain and Nervous System Disorders, and Neurorehabilitation Services
Genolier Swiss Medical Network, Clinique Valmont
CH–1823 Glion/Montreux (Switzerland)
Tel. +41 21 962 3700, Fax +41 21 962 3838, E-Mail jbogousslavsky@valmontgenolier.ch

Bogousslavsky J, Hennerici MG, Bäzner H, Bassetti C (eds): Neurological Disorders in Famous Artists – Part 3. Front Neurol Neurosci. Basel, Karger, 2010, vol 27, pp 46–60

··········· ············

Egon Schiele and Dystonia

Frank J. Erbguth

Department of Neurology, Nuremberg Municipal Academic Hospital, Nuremberg, Germany

---

Abstract

Egon Schiele was a leading Austrian Expressionist painter who, after the era of Gustav Klimt, strongly influenced the artistic scene in Vienna in the early 20th century. Schiele's depiction of his body in his self-portraits in a twisted, contorted, dystonia-like pose raised questions about the possibility of his suffering from dystonia. However, there are no grounds whatsoever for such a hypothesis. Schiele's conception of distorted, at times bizarre, body postures reflects a concourse of the Expressionist formal style of displaying extroverted emotions and psychic conflicts with the emerging perception of photographs of patients with movement disorders in Vienna's art scene and intellectual circles. There are reliable indications that Schiele knew the images of diseases published in the 'Iconographie Photographique de la Salpetriere' and the later 'Nouvelle Iconographie de la Salpetriere' including hysterical and dystonic postures. The brevity of Schiele's life adds to the popular fantasy of the outlaw who lived fast and died young. In fact, however, his drawings sold well to discerning collectors, and his exhibitions were a financial success, so the myth of Schiele as a sacrificial outcast does not tell the whole story. It may be speculated that the figuration of the pathological body in Schiele's self-portraiture was part of modernist strategizing.

Copyright © 2010 S. Karger AG, Basel

Egon Schiele (1890–1918) was a major figurative painter of the early 20th century and is regarded together with Oskar Kokoschka as the leading representative of Austrian Expressionism. Schiele's promising career was cut short by his sudden death from the Spanish influenza at the age of 28. His complete oeuvre encompasses 245 paintings and about 2,000 drawings, gouaches and watercolors. Schiele's many self-portraits and some of his portraits show distorted postures of various body parts evocative of dystonic movement disorders (fig. 1, 2). Due to the fact that Schiele is also shown in a photograph from 1910 with his head in a laterocollis-like position (fig. 3), the question was raised as to whether Schiele himself might have been suffering from dystonia – in particular from

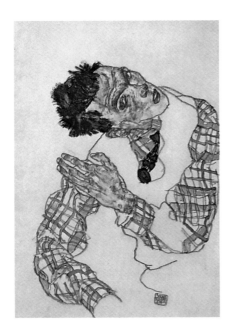

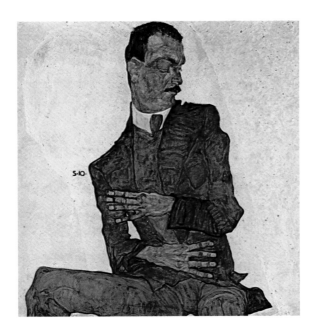

Fig. 1. Self-Portrait with Plaid Shirt. Charcoal and covering color (1917). Card from Welz Gallery Editors, Salzburg, with kind permission.

Fig. 2. Portrait of the art critic Arthur Roessler. Oil on canvas (1910). ©Collection Wien Museum, Vienna, with kind permission.

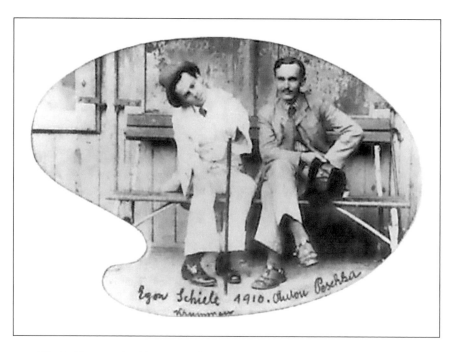

Fig. 3. Photograph of Egon Schiele (left) and Anton Peschka (1910) by Erwin Osen. Private collection.

spasmodic torticollis [Goetz et al., 2001]. However, there are no conclusive biographical sources or indications from contemporary witnesses that would support such a hypothesis. Schiele's dystonic body sculptures and his contorted poses in photographs are to be interpreted rather as a gesture of Expressionist body language [Comini, 1974; Natter und Trummer, 2006]. Though there are interesting indications that Schiele, while not suffering from dystonia himself, was inspired by the photographic images of neurological movement abnormalities, such as hysterical, dystonic or disfigured movements or postures displayed in the journal 'Iconographie Photographique de la Salpêtrière' or in the succeeding publication 'Nouvelle Iconographie de la Salpêtrière: Clinique des Maladies du Systeme Nerveux'. The photographic documents of distorted and dystonic bodies were circulated throughout Europe and were also seen by the intellectual community in Vienna at the time of Sigmund Freud's psychoanalytic concepts. From this point of view, the dystonic gestures of Schiele's portraits and self-portraits reflects on the one hand a stylistic element of Expressionism and, on the other hand, a medically influenced form of perception and exhibition of the human body which was en vogue in Vienna in the early 20th century [Blackshaw, 2007].

Biographical Sketch

Egon Leo Adolf Schiele was born in the Austrian town of Tulln on the River Danube on June 12, 1890, as the fourth child of the stationmaster Adolf Eugen Schiele and his wife Marie. Schiele started his education at the primary school in Tulln, after which he attended the junior secondary school in Krems and then the senior secondary school in Klosterneuburg, where his arts teacher K.L. Strauch recognized and fostered Schiele's artistic talent [Fischer, 1998]. When Schiele was 15 years old, his father died of syphilis, and he became a ward of his maternal uncle, Leopold Czihaczec, who became distressed by Schiele's lack of interest in academic studies, yet recognized his passion and talent for art. In 1906 Schiele applied for admission to the School of Arts and Crafts in Vienna, where Gustav Klimt had once studied. During his first year there, in 1906 at the age of 16, Schiele was sent, at the insistence of several faculty members, to the more traditional Academy of Arts in Vienna. Incidentally, Adolf Hitler was rejected by the Academy in 1907, which has led to a misconception that Schiele and Hitler knew each other in Vienna. Schiele, who studied painting and drawing, sought out Gustav Klimt for support. Klimt generously mentored younger artists, and he took a particular interest in the gifted young Schiele, buying his drawings, offering to exchange them for some of his own, arranging models for him and introducing him to potential patrons. Gustav Klimt introduced Schiele to the 'Wiener Werkstätte', the arts and crafts workshop connected with the 'Secession'. In 1908 Schiele had his first exhibition in Klosterneuburg. Already during his school education he had opposed authoritarian educational standards and boring content of teaching. His school achievements were less important to him than his passion for drawing and painting. Schiele was frustrated by the rigid and conservative academic attitude of his art professor Christian Griepenkerl and left the Academy after only two years. Together with some of his fellow students he formed the Viennese 'Neukunstgruppe' ('New Art Group'). Schiele's opinionated style displeased Griepenkerl to such an extent that he taunted his student, saying 'You have been shit into my class by the devil!' [Nebehay, 1993; Schmidt, 1998].

Schiele achieved a first success in 1909 with the exhibition of his works in the 'Great Vienna Art Exposition', where he encountered the work of Edvard Munch, Jan Toorop and Vincent van Gogh among others. Once free of the constraints of the Academy's conventions, Schiele began to explore not only the human form, but also human sexuality. At that time, many found the explicitness of his works disturbing. Besides artists such as Gustav Klimt and Oskar Kokoschka, Schiele was able to make a name for himself especially with the art critic Arthur Roessler, who supported Schiele through his excellent contacts to the Viennese art scene and played a crucial role in Schiele's further career. Through Roessler's intervention Schiele got to know the art collectors Carl Reininghaus and Dr. Oskar Reichel, who assured financial means for his entry into the Viennese art scene and art market and supplied him with numerous commissions [Natter und Storch, 2004].

The essential turning point of Schiele's career took place in 1910, when the 'enfant terrible' of the Viennese art scene broke once and for all with the elegant decorative painting of art nouveau ('Jugendstil') and increasingly used the stylistic devices of Expressionism [Leopold, 2008; Nebehay, 1993].

In 1911, Schiele met the 17-year-old Valerie (Wally) Neuzil, who lived with him in Vienna and sat as his model for some of his most striking paintings. Very little is known of her, except that she had previously modeled for Gustav Klimt and may have been one of his mistresses. Schiele and Wally wanted to escape what they perceived as the claustrophobic Viennese milieu and went to the small town of Krumau, the birthplace of Schiele's mother. Despite Schiele's family connections in Krumau, he and his lover were driven out of the town by the residents who strongly disapproved of their lifestyle, including his alleged employment of the town's teenage girls as models. Together with Wally, Schiele moved to Neulengbach, 35 km west of Vienna, to find new inspirational surroundings and an inexpensive studio. As it had been in Vienna, Schiele's painting studio became a gathering place for Neulengbach's delinquent children. Schiele's way of life aroused much animosity among the town's inhabitants, and in April 1912 he was arrested for seducing a young girl below the age of consent. At his studio, the police confiscated more than a hundred drawings which they considered pornographic. Schiele was imprisoned while awaiting his trial. The judge dropped the charges of seduction and abduction, but found Schiele guilty of exhibiting erotic drawings in a place accessible to children. In court, the judge burned one of the offending drawings over a candle flame. The 21 days Schiele had already spent in custody were taken into account, and he was sentenced to only 3 days imprisonment. While in prison, Schiele created a series of 12 paintings depicting the difficulties and discomfort of being locked in a jail cell [Kuhl, 2006; Steiner, 1999].

In 1912, Schiele returned to Vienna and was able to reestablish himself, supported by his patron and fatherly friend Gustav Klimt. Schiele also wrote some literary contributions: in 1914 some of his poems were published in the weekly journal 'Die Fackel' ('The Torch') and until 1916 he contributed various theoretical and literary texts to the journal 'Die Aktion' ('The Action') in Berlin. In 1913, the Hans Goltz Gallery, Munich, mounted Schiele's first solo exhibition. Another solo show of his work took place in Paris in 1914 [Kallir, 1998, 2003; Nebehay, 1993].

In 1914, Schiele first glimpsed the sisters Edith and Adéle Harms, whose Protestant middle-class family lived across the street from his studio in the Viennese suburb of Hietzing. In 1915, Schiele chose to marry Edith, but had apparently expected to maintain his relationship with Wally Neuzil. However, Wally left him immediately and never saw him again. Three days after his wedding on June 17, 1915, Schiele was ordered to report for service in the army. There, Schiele was treated well by officers who respected his artistic talent. He was never involved in any fighting at the front and therefore was able to continue painting and sketching while carrying out light guard duties [Artinger, 2001].

Schiele was invited to participate in the 49th exhibition of the Viennese 'Secession' in 1918. Fifty works had been accepted for this exhibition and were displayed in the main hall. Schiele's poster for the exhibition was reminiscent of the Last Supper, with a portrait of himself in the place of Christ. The show was a triumphant success and, as a result, prices for Schiele's drawings increased.

After the death of Gustav Klimt in 1918, Egon Schiele meanwhile had ascended to the position of the leading exponent of the Expressionist avant-garde of Vienna. Unfortunately, the year of the end of World War I was also the year of Schiele's death. In 1918 the Spanish influenza pandemic, which claimed 20 million lives in Europe, reached Vienna. On October 19, 1918, Schiele's wife Edith, who was 6 months pregnant, fell ill with the flu and succumbed to the disease on October 28. Schiele died only 3 days after his wife on the day when she was buried. He was 28 years old. During the 3 days between their deaths, Schiele drew a few sketches of Edith on her sickbed; these were his last works [Schröder, 1997].

Schiele's Works

Schiele's work is famous worldwide and noted for the many portraits of others as well as himself and nude drawings. He also painted tributes to Van Gogh's Sunflowers as well as landscapes and still lives. The twisted, grotesque body shapes of his self-portraits, the erotic aura of his nude paintings and the expressive lines that characterize Schiele's paintings and drawings mark the artist as an early exponent of Expressionism, although at the beginning of his career he was still strongly associated with the art nouveau movement

('Jugendstil') [Müller-Tamm, 1995]. The largest and most important collection of Schiele's work is housed in the Leopold Museum in Vienna. Schiele's bizarre, dystonia-like compositions of the human body allow two possible interpretations and explanations. The first is that Schiele utilized dystonic movements and postures as stylistic elements of Expressionism without any allusion to the really existing movement disorders and a medical context of pathological disfigurement. The second is that Schiele's style represents a strategic and astute awareness of the taste of the art market [Blackshaw, 2007]. This taste was influenced by the fascinating and esoteric medical photographs of the 'Iconographie' journals of the hospital for mental diseases in Paris, La Salpêtrire [Didi-Huberman, 1997].

Dystonic Postures as a Stylistic Element of Expressionism

The model Schiele mostly used was himself. The painter does not emphasize outward conditions of physical existence, but works on penetrating into his being. Schiele, as compared to his contemporaries, breaks with tradition most radically as far as esthetic appearance is concerned and prefers artistic finding of the truth in an expressionistic, figurative sense. In his drawings and paintings he used all the possibilities of facial and physical expression to the point of bizarre postures and distortions. But also in photography, he works with an expressionistic gesture and arranges extraordinary body poses and movements. For example, in a photograph from 1910 showing Schiele together with his friend Anton Peschka, he poses with his head in a position as it is known in dystonic laterocollis. This photo was the origin for speculations that Schiele could have suffered from cervical dystonia. However, there are no sources, indications or reports from himself or from contemporary witnesses to support the theory that the artist suffered from dystonic disease. The small excerpt of some of his portraits is part of its quality of meaning; often the head is cut off shortly above the forehead. The subjects painted – mostly Schiele himself – communicate with the observer: On the one hand, a relationship between the observer and the artist is established with the help of the latter's eye contact; on the other hand, communication is often interrupted by a dystonia-like grimace or rejecting gesture. Schiele's self-portraits are interpreted as not resulting from contemplating his own soul, but as stemming from turning his immediate feelings outward in an active, often exaggerated way and thus demonstrating various possibilities of self-perception [Fischer, 1998]. Thus, Schiele's understanding of physical expression resembles to some extent Sigmund Freud's concept of 'conversion', which the Viennese neurologist and later psychoanalyst developed during his research stay with the famous

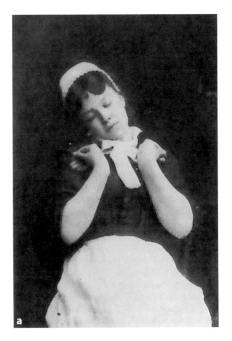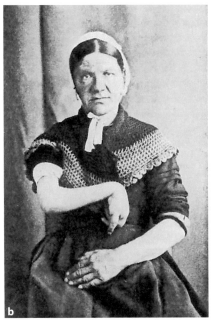

Fig. 4. Photographs from the 'Iconographie photographique de La Salpêtrière'. *a* 'Augustine', Planche XIII [Bourneville and Régnard, 1879]. *b* 'Josephine Delet', Planche III [Bourneville and Régnard, 1878]. Photographs kindly provided by the Bibliotheque Charcot, UPMC – Université Pierre et Marie Curie, Hôpital de la Salpêtrière, Paris.

French neurologist Jean Martin Charcot in Paris in 1885 [Blackshaw, 2007; Didi-Huberman, 1997]. Freud interpreted the bizarre body postures and movements of hysteria as expressions of internal psychic conflicts which are turned outward (fig. 4).

From the traditional viewpoint of interpreting Schiele's work, he utilizes the expressiveness of the human body by using gestures and dystonic deformations as a simile. The position and motion of the hands in an expressive, unreal gesture are interpreted to be a symbol of communication at a standstill. By means of habitual distortions the subject of the self-portrait becomes a stranger to the painter, and so he even sees himself as someone else would see him. Therefore Schiele plays with different roles and puts on masks, such as monk, prophet or saint [Fischer, 1998; Nebehay, 1993].

Even the last photo of Schiele on his deathbed shows him in an arranged, unusual posture with his arms and hands twisted: his left behind his head and his right across his chest (fig. 5).

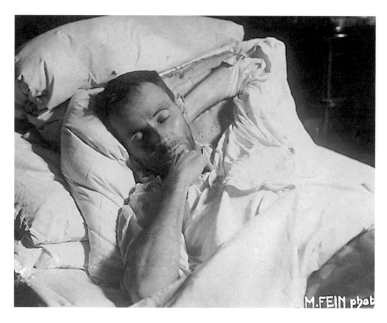

Fig. 5. Photograph of Schiele on his deathbed. Photograph by Martha Fein (1918). ©Albertina collection, Vienna, with kind permission.

The Neurologically Diseased Body as Source and Inspiration for Schiele's 'Dystonic' Figuration

The interpretation explaining Schiele's body distortion exclusively as an expression of a traumatized individual who used the self-portrait as a means of articulating emotions in an expressionistic manner might negate the influence of the cultural context in Vienna at the turn of the century. Other interpretations argue that Schiele's turn to this particular genre, style and esthetics at that particular moment was a strategic move, showing his astute awareness of market taste and dynamics. Gemma Blackshaw [2007] suggests that Schiele's body interpretation was not primarily an 'inward-looking' art practice, but rather a practice that was geared specifically towards a commercial local art market. The questions as to what made this kind of self-portrait or portrait so marketable and where the new gesture of the body came from are answered by Blackshaw with the reference to a common iconography of Schiele's painted bodies and the photographs of patients suffering from diseases of the nervous system, published in Paris-based neuropathology journals which circulated in

Vienna. The journals provided Schiele with a new vocabulary of the body which could be used powerfully to underscore – in a truly modernist fashion – his 'suffering' and therefore his 'genius'. Cultivation of such an identity was crucial amongst a group of patrons tired of the artist-collective ideology of Secession culture and keen to promote young men representing the 'new blood' – for which there were many contenders. The fact that Schiele's peers and competitors, such as Oskar Kokoschka and Max Oppenheimer, made similar use of this iconography of the body, speedily working it into their own portrait portfolios, shows how aware this group of young men were of its appeal to their patrons.

Klaus Albrecht Schröder [1997] pointed to photographic journals popularizing nervous disorder as possible sources for Schiele's self-representation, concentrating on the striking iconographic parallels. Schröder took his examples from the 'Iconographie Photographique de la Salpêtrière' journal, which was produced in three volumes from 1876 to 1880 under the direction of Jean-Martin Charcot at the Paris hospital for diseases of the nervous system, La Salpêtrière, and circulated widely throughout Europe. The journal concentrated on the various manifestations of hysteria – a condition deemed more common in women than in men – which was typified by bizarre body postures, hallucinations and a susceptibility to hypnosis. The allure of the journal lay in its photographic documentation of the female body when released – via hypnosis, the inhalation of vapors or the pressing of hystereogenic zones of the body – from its civilizing bonds of bourgeois behavior. Photographs sensationally captured female patients in the midst of attacks, convulsing in their hospital beds. The violence of the attacks recorded, the voyeuristic appeal of watching the body as it moved through hysterical sequences or 'attitudes passionnelles', and the bewildering array of patient responses (such as limb contracture or reenactments of the crucifixion) made the image of the hysteric a popular one [Didi-Huberman, 1997]. The popularity of the 'Iconographie Photographique' is underlined by the fact that the Salpêtrière team produced a succeeding journal between 1888 and 1918 under the new title 'Nouvelle Iconographie de la Salpêtrière: Clinique des Maladies du Système Nerveux'. This later journal – separated from its predecessor by a period of 8 years – moved the focus away from hysteria to neurological disease as signaled in both the male and female body. Photographs of fibrous skin growths and spinal deformity, conditions that were included under the umbrella of neuropathology, are perhaps not – initially – as interesting as the dramatic gendering and eroticizing of hysteria we see performed in the first journal editions. The 'Nouvelle Iconographie' journal displayed photographs of predominantly male patients in a canon of the physical extremes of the body in pain. Blackshaw [2007] refers to obvious similarities between a series of medical

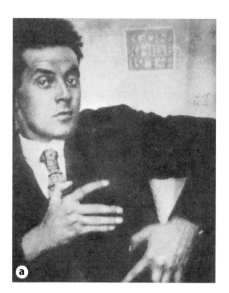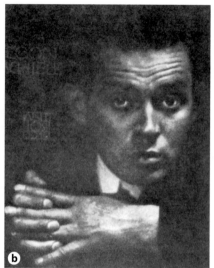

Fig. 6. Photographs of Egon Schiele by Anton Josef Trcka (1914). ©Albertina collection, Vienna, with kind permission.

photographs entitled 'Macrodactylie', in which close-up shots of the fronts and backs of disfigured hands are displayed, and the configuration of hand positions in Schiele's paintings and photographic self-portraits [Bégouin and Sabrazés 1901; Blackshaw, 2007; Lejars 1903] (fig. 6–8), Klaus-Albrecht Schröder [1997] characterizes the role of the French photographic medical journals for Egon Schiele as 'a quarry of motives which do not symbolize rationality, arrangement and control, but expressiveness and authenticity of the psyche and of the emotions'.

The discussion of new medical and psychological aspects of neurological and psychiatric diseases was considered to be a matter of public interest, with Vienna's new psychiatric spaces being opened up to the view of the 'outside world'. For example, an exhibition on the care of the insane was opened to mark the Emperor Franz Josef I's Silver Jubilee celebrations in 1898, which polarized the traditional approach to psychiatric treatment (using objects such as shackled wax figures) with the contemporary (represented by models of newly built observation wards). The patient's body became – in many ways – a public body, to be reassuringly displayed to audiences. Artistic interventions from Vienna's modernist circles in the care and cure of psychiatric patients were well rehearsed by individuals working in the same circles as Schiele before

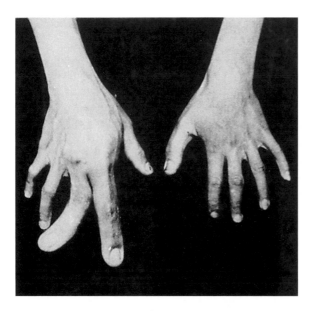

Fig. 7. Photograph of a case of macrodactyly in the 'Nouvelle Iconographie de La Salpêtrière', table XVI, Planche VIII [Lejars, 1903]. Photograph kindly provided by the Bibliotheque Charcot, UPMC – Université Pierre et Marie Curie, Hôpital de la Salpêtrière, Paris.

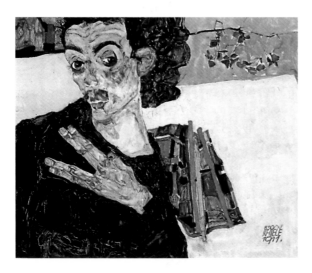

Fig. 8. Self-Portrait with Black Vase. Oil on wood (1911). ©Collection Wien Museum, Vienna, with kind permission.

he turned to an iconography of pathology in 1910. Schiele also had access to images of the pathological body.

Schiele's friend, the pathological anatomist and gynecologist Dr Erwin von Graff, gave him permission to draw the patients at the gynecological university hospital in 1910. The university hospital championed the pathological anatomy approach to psychiatry and held the complete edition of the 'Nouvelle Iconographie'. In exactly the same year, Schiele embraced the image of the diseased body. It therefore can be hypothesized that he translated the new iconography to which he had access at the University into his self-portrait practice. Another friend of Schiele's, the theater painter and mime artist Erwin Dominik Osen, who called himself 'Mime van' Osen (1891–1970), wrote a letter to him in 1913 in which he states: 'I still have to finish a portrait in Vienna and a few drawings at Steinhof (= Psychiatric Hospital) for the "Science Day" where Dr. Kronfeld will be speaking on pathological expression in portraiture. ... I am already simulating all diseases so that I may get away sooner'. This text is proof of Schiele's exposure to ideas on the representation of pathology in portraiture. Not only was Schiele working closely with Osen as an artist who was drawing patients, he was also meeting a doctor whose interest lay in pathological expression [Blackshaw, 2007].

Without doubt, there are iconographic links between Schiele's self-portraits and the photographs of patients with abnormal body postures and diseased gestures. According to Blackshaw's hypothesis, Schiele's consultation of the photographs – readily available in Vienna's medical and public libraries – was a canny move by an artist who was aware of current debate in Vienna about neuropathology and the debilitating effects of modern life on the body, as well as the inadequacy of Secessionist style of art to represent this body. Schiele was certainly helped in this endeavor, and one should not underestimate the role of physician friends working in pathological anatomy, critics such as Roessler who championed the skin-peeling techniques of the new 'Young Viennese Painters', and patrons such as Reininghaus who purchased the self-portrait that first presented the stylistic maneuver to a modern, avant-garde expression of the human body. Blackshaw speculates that the iconography of pathology was proffered and fostered not mainly by the artist, but by his market. She considers Schiele's way of painting bodies as a collaborative effort, with Schiele presenting his body as a pathological and pitiful site for male spectators who could – in looking, buying, exchanging and identifying – promote the artist as the 'precociously diseased' young Vienna.

Schiele's Life and Work in Literature and Film

Schiele's life and work have been the subject of contributions in literature and film. Mario Vargas Llosa uses the work of Schiele as a conduit to seduce and morally exploit the main character Alfonso ('Fonchito') in his 1997 novel 'The Notebooks of Don Rigoberto' [Llosa, 1997]. Schiele has also been the subject of a 1980 German biographical film, 'Egon Schiele: Excess & Punishment', directed by Herbert Vesely with Mathieu Carriere as Egon Schiele, Jane Birkin as his early artistic muse, and Christine Kaufman as his wife. There is also a film 'Klimt' from 2006 directed by Raoul Ruiz with John Malkovich as Gustav Klimt in which Egon Schiele (acted by Nikolai Kinski) plays an important role. Jamie Tanner [2002] dedicated his comic 'The perpetual child' to the biography of Egon Schiele. In 1995, Stephan Mazurek presented a theatrical dance production called 'Egon Schiele', for which Rachel's, an American post-rock group, composed a score titled 'Music for Egon Schiele'.

References

Artinger K: Minikunstführer Egon Schiele. Cologne, Könemann, 2001.

Bégouin P, Sabrazés J: Macrodactylie et microdaclylie. Nouvelle iconographie de la Salpêtrière Paris 1901;4:305–315.

Blackshaw G: The pathological body: modernist strategising in Egon Schiele's self-portraiture. Oxford Art J 2007;30:377–401.

Bourneville DM, Régnard P: Observation III in: Iconographie Photographique de La Salpetriere. 1878;2:22–30.

Bourneville DM, Régnard P: Observation XII in: Iconographie Photographique de La Salpetriere. 1879;3:187–199.

Comini A: Egon Schiele's Portraits. Berkeley, University of California Press, 1974.

Didi-Huberman G: Die Erfindung der Hysterie. Die photographische Klinik von Jean-Martin Charcot. Munich, Wilhelm Fink, 1997.

Fischer WG: Egon Schiele. 1890–1918. Pantomimen der Lust. Visionen der Sterblichkeit. Cologne, Taschen, 1998.

Goetz C, Chmura TA, Lanska DJ: History of dystonia. Part 4. Mov Disord 2001;16:339–345.

Kallir J: Egon Schiele. The Complete Works. Including a Biography and a Catalogue raisonne. Expanded edition, New York, Harry N. Abrams, 1998.

Kallir J: Egon Schiele. Drawings and Watercolours. London, Thames & Hudson, 2003.

Kuhl I: Egon Schiele. Munich, Prestel Verlag, 2006.

Lejars F: Un fait de macrodactylie. Nouvelle iconographie de la Salpêtrière Paris 1903;1:37–40.

Leopold E, Leopold Museum Wien (eds): Der Lyriker Egon Schiele. Munich, Leopold Museum/Prestel, 2008.

Llosa MV: The Notebooks of Don Rigoberto. New York, Penguin Books, 1997.

Müller-Tamm P (ed): Egon Schiele. Inszenierung und Identität. Cologne, Dumont, 1995.

Natter TG, Storch U (eds): Schiele & Roessler. Der Künstler und sein Förderer. Kunst und Networking im frühen 20. Jahrhundert. Ostfildern-Ruit, Hatje Cantz, 2004.

Natter TG, Trummer T: Die Tafelrunde. Egon Schiele und sein Kreis. Meisterwerke des österreichischen Frühexpressionismus. Cologne, DuMont, 2006.

Nebehay CM: Egon Schiele. Leben und Werk in Dokumenten und Bildern. Munich, Deutscher Taschenbuchverlag, 1983.

Schmidt R: Das Enfant terrible wollte die innere Wahrheit zum Ausdruck bringen. Ärztezeitung 1998;197:23–24.

Schröder KA: Zu Egon Schieles Darstellung dissoziierter Bewusstseinszustände; in Brugger I, Gorsen P, Schröder KA (eds): Kunst & Wahn. Vienna, Kunstforum Wien/Cologne, Dumont 1997.

Steiner R: Schiele. Die Mitternachtsseele eines Künstlers, Cologne, Taschen, 1999.

Tanner J: The Perpetual Child. Biography of Painter Egon Schiele. SPX 2002 Anthology; www.jami-etanner.com

Prof. Dr. Frank Joachim Erbguth
Department of Neurology, Nuremberg Municipal Academic Hospital
Breslauer Strasse 201
DE–90471 Nürnberg (Germany)
Tel. +49 911 398 2491, Fax +49 911 398 3164, E-Mail erbguth@klinikum-nuernberg.de

Bogousslavsky J, Hennerici MG, Bäzner H, Bassetti C (eds): Neurological Disorders in Famous Artists – Part 3. Front Neurol Neurosci. Basel, Karger, 2010, vol 27, pp 61–83

······················

Syphilis in German-Speaking Composers – 'Examination Results Are Confidential'

H. Bäzner[a,b], *M.G. Hennerici*[a]

[a]Department of Neurology, Universitätsmedizin Mannheim, University of Heidelberg, Mannheim, [b]Neurologische Klinik, Klinikum Stuttgart, Bürgerhospital, Stuttgart, Germany

---

Abstract

Syphilis was endemic in Europe in the 19th century. Therefore, infection with the disease was common. As far as can be determined from contemporary sources, Schubert, Schumann and Wolf all died from the consequences of syphilis. However, as families tried to keep the shameful secret, the original sources are sparse. In this article, we will briefly illustrate Schubert's case and will then focus on Robert Schumann and Hugo Wolf. Both shared such a variety of symptoms that interfered with their artistic expression, especially in respect to Lied compositions, that it seems improbable that they should have suffered from different diagnoses, as has been argued previously.

Neurosyphilis was endemic in 19th century, an effective cure not being available. At that time treatment was largely based on only moderately effective mercury preparations, these, however, were associated with severe side effects. Although neurology as a discipline made enormous progress in the 19th century and the diagnosis of neurosyphilis could be made clinically with great certainty, the infectious agent of *Treponema pallidum* and Paul Ehrlich's salvarsan treatment were only discovered in the first decade of the 20th century. As a consequence, the disease remained a threat to sexually active people [Singh and Romanowski, 1999].

Syphilis was perceived to be a consequence of immoral, improper, or promiscuous sexuality; the diagnosis resulting in severe social stigmatization. This fact most probably led to many historical medical analyses being incomplete or misleading. Today the diagnosis of syphilis in these geniuses remains not unanimously accepted by experts in the field of musical and medical history.

Naturally, syphilis in Franz Schubert, Robert Schumann and Hugo Wolf cannot be confirmed retrospectively using modern diagnostic tools. At the beginning of the 21st century, however, in large part made possible by the publication of Robert Schumann's medical records [Franken, 1997a, b; Mayeda et al., 2006]– and the striking similarities with Hugo Wolf's case [Franken 1997a], we postulate that the diagnosis of syphilis in both composers can be made with reasonable certainty. Schubert at least seems to have been treated for the suspected disease, his case however being different in that he never progressed to the form of tertiary neurosyphilis [Hetenyi 1986].

Characteristically, in all the three composers, euphoric surges of creative energy, associated with emotional highs, produced clusters of productivity resulting in quite phenomenal series of song composition.

The age of romanticism, stressing at times banked emotion as a source of experience, was probably the perfect environment to nurture the esthetics typical for poems and music of the time. It remains speculative if this elated 'sensitivity' compensated for the often unfulfilled dreams and wishes.

Franz Schubert (1797–1828) – Legends and Truth

Schubert (fig. 1) is so famous that a special note on his character is certainly redundant for the purpose of this chapter. Of course, many myths regarding his personality have been handed down until today, for instance that this small and gross person was always surrounded by a corona of friends and admirers. We have the picture in mind of the gay piano player with the curly hair and thick glasses whose shyness was such an impediment for an amorous affaire that he never married. As to his final illness, there is debate about a possible diagnosis of *Typhus abdominalis*, although the contemporary diagnosis of 'Nervenfieber' and the available sources do not support this idea. More convincingly, his first serious illness leading to a chronic ailment can be diagnosed with reasonable certainty as syphilis [Hetenyi 1986; Sams, 1980; Franken, 1989; Deutsch, 1921/1922; Böhme, 1987; Kerner, 1998; Solomon, 1989].

Hugo Wolf (1860–1903) – Biographical Notes and Personality Traits

One of his closest friends, Edmund Hellmer, introduced Hugo Wolf (fig. 2) as follows: 'He was of very short stature (154 cm) – broad shoulders, strong and short his neck –his small hands and feet being almost graceful. His head slightly bent forward – face and hands colored like old ivory [...] his eyes were dark like black-ink spots and seemed to burn from an inner fire. His short-cut hair was

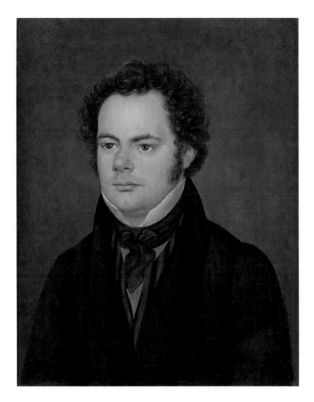

Fig. 1. Franz Schubert. Canvas 1828, artist unknown, previously attributed to Joseph Mähler. According to new sources painted by Anton Depauly [Schirlbauer, 2004]. Gesellschaft der Musikfreunde, Vienna, with kind permission.

smooth and blond, his beard on lips and chin brownish [...] his clothes were modest but always perfectly clean [...] scrupulous order is the principle of his life' [Hellmer, 1921]. Wolf's most important biographer, Frank Walker [1960], documented some remarkable 'Conversations with Hugo Wolf', which nicely characterize the composer. His judgment on women's role in society is all but legendary: 'However, the woman must naturally always preserve decorum'. On another occasion, he displayed rather rude behavior. Having laid down on a sofa and resting in the house of friends: 'I'm quite indifferent. I do what I please. If people don't like it, they should say so. All responsibility for my conduct I take on myself.' According to Robert Hernried [1945], 'Wolf was both tough and gentle, overbearing and humble, intellectually acute and naively child-like, condemnatory and forgiving, a Titan and a humble mortal. His fiery tempera-

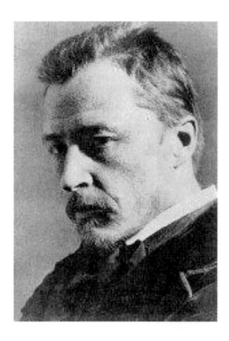

Fig. 2. Hugo Wolf, 1895.

ment went from one extreme to the other, and all too often it must have been incomprehensible to bourgeois stodginess and complacency.'

Wolf was born in Windischgraz which then belonged to the Austrian Empire and is now a small town in Slovenia called Slovenj Gradec. He was a very bad student except for musical studies, and was dismissed from several secondary schools as well as from the Vienna Conservatory due to lack of discipline. For most of his life, Wolf stayed in Vienna. He changed apartments on numerous occasions, having complained about the noise of others [Walker, 1968; Werba, 1971; Decsey, 1903–1906; Dorschel, 1985; Hanolka, 1988; Newman, 1966].

Wolf's activities as a critic for the Vienna 'Salonblatt' began to pick up in the 1880s. He was quite merciless in his criticism but fervent in his support of the genius of Liszt, Schubert, and Chopin. His most famous victim was Johannes Brahms. The intensity and expressive strength of his convictions made him numerous enemies in musical Vienna [Walker, 1968; Werba, 1971]. His judgment on the late works by Robert Schumann was strict at best: '[Schumann's] "Faust" is very weak, except for a few passages in the third part. All his later things get feebler and have almost no substance. I am no great lover of his symphonies either. Only in a small frame, in miniature style, there he is a master' [Walker, 1960]. If we agree with this statement, we have also to admit that Wolf himself had great difficulty in composing works of the 'large frame'. The 'Rosé Quartet' would not even look at his only string quartet after having been criticized in one of his regular columns. On another occasion, at the rehearsal of novelties, his tone poem of Penthesilea was met by the Vienna Philharmonic Orchestra under conductor Hans Richter with nothing but derision for the man who had dared to criticize Brahms [Walker, 1960].

Robert Schumann (1810–1856) – Brief Note on His Personality

Robert Schumann's biography is very well known [Boucourechliev, 1958; von Wasielewski, 1906], therefore we will only focus on some details of his personality. He was quite tall, walked slowly, dragging his feet, at times tip-toeing. Contemporaries mentioned that he often kept his eyes almost closed, leading to speculation that he may have had reduced vision. According to his first biographer, Joseph von Wasielewsky [1906], Schumann 'lacked the ability to put himself in close rapport with others, and to make his meaning clear to them; this was because he either was silent, or spoke so low that he could not be understood'. Especially in his younger years he was known to drink alcohol, at times excessively, and smoked cigars for many years.

The Infection

The first definite mention of Schubert's illness can be found in 1823. In a letter of February 28, he writes to the Hofrath von Mosel, that his physical condition still does not allow him to leave his house [Deutsch, 1964]. An earlier letter to the same person is lost. Hence, we do not know the exact onset and the duration of the illness and closer details regarding his physical condition and of his inability to leave the house. According to Deutsch [1921/1922], he was hospitalized for a period of time in the General Hospital in Vienna, possibly in May and June of 1823, where he wrote a deeply depressive poem speaking of 'deep longing seeks to attain finer worlds', asking for a 'deliverance from profound pains', he describes his life as of 'vulnerable to unspeakable depression', 'approaching its eternal demise'. Possibly, parts of the Liederzyklus 'Die schöne Müllerin' may have been composed in the hospital. Wilhelm von Chézy, the son of Schubert's Rosamunde librettist Hermina von Chézy, wrote in 1863 that Schubert 'had strayed into those wrong paths which generally admit of no return, at least of no healthy one' and added that 'the charming "Müllerlieder" were composed under sufferings of a quite different kind from those immortalized in the music which he put into the mouth of the poor lovelorn miller lad' [Solomon, 1989]. Most biographers cite Deutsch [1964] with the next available account from Schubert's hand dating from August 14, 1823, when he wrote to Schober that he felt better. He tells Schober that he corresponds regularly with Dr. August von Schaeffer, his physician, but doubts regaining complete health again. As to an exact occasion of a syphilitic infection, there are no convincing sources. Classical and recent biographies speculate about an infection in November 1822 when he moved from Schober's to his own family home in order to seek medical treatment for the infectious stage of the disease. Some contemporary biographers speculate – kind of sensation-mongering – about Schubert's homosexuality and a possible infection while living with Johann Mayrhofer in 1821 [Solomon, 1989]. In conclusion, 'there is no indication as to whether the act which brought on Schubert's illness was a homosexual or heterosexual one' [Newbould, 1999].

Wolf's musical gift and his charm earned him attention and patronage as soon as he was introduced to Vienna society as a very young man. Decisively, in his early Vienna days he was most probably infected with syphilis. If we take the memoirs of Alma Mahler at face value, 'Hugo Wolf as a very young man (17 years old) was taken by Adalbert Goldschmidt into the so-called "Lehmgrube" (a brothel) where Goldschmidt played dance music, for which he was often "awarded" with a young woman without charge. He presented his "honorarium" once to his friend Wolf, and Wolf took away with him "the wound that never will heal"' [Mahler, 1940].

With respect to the infection in Robert Schumann's case, an episode noted in his diaries is important [Eismann and Nauhaus, 1971–1987]. Schumann had a sexual relationship with a woman named 'Christel'. Schumann also called her 'Charitas' and meticulously noted and counted their rendezvous. On May 12, 1831, he speaks of a 'bad wound' that caused 'biting and devouring pains'. His friend and medical student Glock 'made an embarrassed face'. Schumann expressed his hope that 'only guilt brings Nemesis' and speaks of his 'incautiousness'. On June 4, the remark of 'the frenulum bitten by daffodil water' may indicate medical treatment of the primary syphilitic lesion. Many years later one can find the following entry in his diary: 'Troubled year 1836: Sought out Charitas and consequences thereof in January 1837'. This can be interpreted as a document of Schumann's growing anxiousness with respect to the potential sequels of his earlier adventure.

Some authors have argued against the diagnosis of syphilis, referring to the fact that Robert and Clara Schumann (fig. 3) had eight children. This argument must be rejected: the infection ('Charitas') dates back to May 1831 and

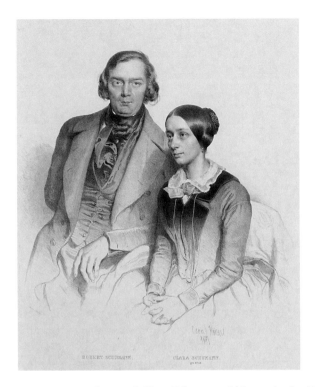

Fig. 3. Robert und Clara Schumann. Lithography by Eduard Kaiser, Vienna 1847. Gesellschaft der Musikfreunde, Vienna, with kind permission.

the marriage of Robert and Clara was on September 12, 1840. Since sexual transmission of *T. pallidum* occurs only when mucocutaneous syphilitic lesions are present and such manifestations are uncommon after the first year of infection, Robert was certainly not infectious given the latency of 9 years after the primary infection.

Productivity in Clusters

1888 and 1889 were amazingly productive years for Hugo Wolf. He travelled to the vacation home of the Werner family in Perchtoldsdorf in order to compose in solitude. Here, at astonishing pace, he produced more than 50 songs after poems by Mörike. Still in the same year, the 'Eichendorff-Lieder' followed, then into 1889 the 51 'Goethe-Lieder'. The 'Spanisches Liederbuch'

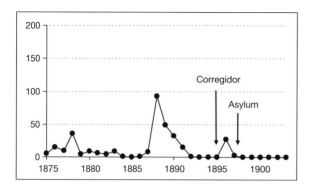

Fig. 4. Creativity in clusters: Hugo Wolf's Lied compositions are clustered in several short periods. Shortly after the composition of his opera 'The Corregidor' in 1895 he produced his last songs.

was begun in October 1889, totaling the number of songs composed in these two years to more than 140. This productiveness is all the more remarkable when considering other phases in Wolf's career (such as 1884–1886 and 1892–1895), when his creativity seemed completely stalled [Walker, 1968; Werba, 1971; Decsey, 1903–1906; Dorschel, 1985; Hanolka, 1988; Newman, 1966] (fig. 4).

Quite interestingly we find the same episodic frenzied working pace in Schumann's oeuvre. In 1840, he composed more than 150 songs, in the years of 1849–1850 more than 100 songs were produced (fig. 5). On October 19, 1840, Clara Schumann notes in the joint diary of the Schumanns': 'Robert says he cannot compose just now, which depresses him. This grieves me very much. Doesn't he remember all he has composed during this last year? Must the mind never rest? Surely it will burst forth later with all the greater power ...' Franz Schubert showed a similar composing pattern. His productive career, however, was considerably shorter and he died 5 years after the first symptoms of syphilis occurred.

Schubert's Disease Course

Schubert's friends informed each other about the disease course in their letters. After a brief phase of reconvalescence following the first symptoms in early 1823, the disease relapsed in autumn 1823. Moritz von Schwind wrote in a letter to Schober dated November 9, 1823 that the friends attended: 'a kind of

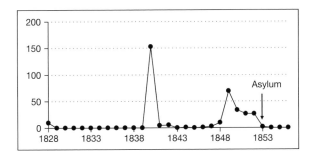

Fig. 5. Creativity in clusters: Robert Schumann's Lied compositions are clustered in several short periods. After admission to the asylum in Endenich he composed no more songs.

bacchanal at the Crown, where we all dined, except Schubert, who was laid up that day' [Deutsch, 1957]. 'Schaeffer and Bernard (Dr. J. Bernhardt, physician in Vienna), who visited him, [...] speak of a 4 week period, after which he might be well again'. Schubert wrote to Schober on November 30, 1823: '[...] I hope to regain my health again, and this [...] will make me forget a lot of sufferings' [Deutsch, 1964]. On December 24, 1823, Schwind wrote to Schober: 'Schubert is better, and it will not be long before he goes about with his own hair again, which had to be shorn owing to the rash. He wears a very cosy wig' [Deutsch, 1957]. An eruption of papular skin rash required hair-shaving, furthermore a strict diet was recommended by Schubert's physician Dr. Bernhardt. On March 6, 1824, again Schwind noticed that 'Schubert [...] said, that some days of the new treatment made him feel, as if the disease was broken and everything was different now' (letter to Schober) [Deutsch, 1957]. There is no further specification of this new treatment. Deeply depressed Schubert wrote to his friend Kupelwieser on March 31, 1824: 'I feel myself to be the most unhappy, the most wretched man in the world [...] each night as I go to sleep, I hope I will not wake up again, and each morning merely proclaims the previous day's grief to me' [Deutsch, 1964]. Later there is an indication of pain in Schubert's left arm, when Schwind wrote to Schober: 'Schubert is unwell. He complains of pain in his left arm, such as he cannot play the piano' [Deutsch, 1957]. More specific, Doblhoff speaks of pain in the bones (letter to Schober April 24, 1824) and adds that Schubert cannot sing [Deutsch, 1957]. Until the beginning of 1826, Schubert was rather well, when Eduard von Bauernfeld placed a brief note in his diary saying that Schubert was sick and therefore unable to attend a dinner at New Year's Eve with Schober [Deutsch, 1957]. A quite interesting remark later on in Bauernfeld's diary has given occasion to speculation. He wrote that 'Schubert [is] half ill' (he requires 'young peacocks' as did Benvenuto Cellini) [Deutsch, 1957]. Benvenuto Cellini, born in 1500, was another famous syphilitic patient, and was known for his love of peacocks as part of his meals. Hence, deciphering Bauernfeld's remark, he seems to allude to the specific nature of Schubert's disease [Solomon, 1989]. On October 27, 1827, Schubert wrote of his common headaches. Later that month, he apologized to Anna Hönig to be unable to attend a dinner party, because 'I am ill, and in a way that totally unfits me for such a gathering'. In the summer of 1828, Schubert complained of vertigo and 'blood flushes' [Deutsch, 1964]. Following the advice of the Hofrat Dr. Ernst Rinna von Sarenbach, Schubert moved from Vienna to his brother Ferdinand who lived in the suburban Neu-Wieden. There, however, he lived no longer than 2 months, never feeling well again.

Regarding this 5- to 6-year period of chronic disease, most authors agree that it was syphilis. Following this hypothesis, Schubert was infected in late 1822 or early 1823. At the time, this disease was common in Vienna and symptoms, including fever, malaise, and a generalized rash, were familiar to all doctors and many laymen too. In this context, Schubert's depressive poem dating from May 1823 may well reflect his sad perspective. If the initial treatment was really done in the large Vienna hospital, Schubert will also have met several patients with the same disease. Following the commonest disease course, the skin rash progresses during the next few months to dome-shaped dull red papules including the face and scalp. Schubert's head was indeed shaved in the summer of 1823 – a treatment usually recommended for hair loss or scabs at that time, both of which may be associated with syphilis in the secondary stage of the disease. His arm pain and loss of voice can also be interpreted in the same direction. Medical treatment of syphilis was largely based on mercury preparations. Detailed indications of mercury use can be found in the writings of Dres. Rinna von Sarenbach and von Vering, both of whom were also treating Schubert during his final illness [Hetenyi, 1986]. Unfortunately, we do not know for sure whether or not Schubert was treated with mercury at this stage of the disease. Remarkably a lot of authentic sources seem to have been destroyed, such as the correspondence with Jenger, Pachler, and Hüttenbrenner. The latter burned the diary he kept about those days. Hence, important details are not available and in part kept secret.

Neurasthenic Prodromal Phase in Schumann and Wolf

After a hopeful start in 1850, Schumann's position as a city music director in Düsseldorf became controversial. In Düsseldorf, Robert and Clara were warmly welcomed and had met a well-drilled, though partly dilettante orchestra. Schumann wrote in a letter to his predecessor Hiller nine months before his arrival in Düsseldorf that he did not 'expect much culture in an orchestra, and [was] prepared to meet common musicians, but not rude or malicious ones' [Hopkins Porter, 1989].

The documents of the growing tensions between the authorities of the musical society and the Schumann family fall in a period that may well be called the prodromal phase of Schumann's final illness. As early as 1851, the executive committee of the General Music Society was alarmed by the fact that a large segment of the public had criticized Schumann's conducting, deploring that he often appeared to be dreaming and was clumsy and slow speaking. Further, discipline in the chorus and orchestra was steadily deteriorating. By the summer of 1852 Schumann's debilitating ill health forced him temporarily to relinquish his conducting duties until early December to Julius Tausch, his deputy [Hopkins Porter, 1989].

By the end of 1852, Deputy Mayor Wortmann remarked that 'the orchestra misses, under Herr Schumann, the solid, sure indication of tempos, even beats, clear, definite, and understandable comments' [Neyses, 1927].

Joseph Wilhelm von Wasielewski (1822–1896), the new concertmaster of the orchestra, reported that Schumann 'lacked the physical energy and endurance requisite for a director: he was always easily exhausted and was obliged to rest at intervals during a rehearsal. Nor did he exercise any sort of care or oversight' [von Wasielewski, 1906].

Also in Hugo Wolf's case a neurasthenic prodromal phase seems likely. While he composed the score of his opera 'The Corregidor' in 1895 he was extremely sensitive to any noise. It is reported that he shot and killed singing birds [Walker, 1968]. Although Wolf had hoped that his opera would have been performed in Vienna, Berlin, or Prague, he had to accept that with the promotion of his good friends in southern Germany 'The Corregidor' was set on stage in Mannheim. During the rehearsals he was unpleasant and spoke of the musicians as 'idiots one cannot work with', and wrote to Melanie Köchert that 'the whole gang [...] was incapable'. Though the premiere was a success, however, only one further performance followed in Mannheim [Hernried, 1940].

Outbreak of General Paresis: Suicidal Attempts and Hospitalization

In contrast to Franz Schubert whose disease began 6 years before his death, both Schumann and Wolf lived much longer after the primary infection. Both reached the stadium of general paresis, while Schubert probably died from meningovascular syphilis. Wolf's final illness stage began at the latest in summer 1897, when he intended to accompany his friend Haberlandt on a bicycle tour. For this purpose, he took bicycle-riding lessons in June 1897 which had to be stopped due to severe coordination deficits. Wolf was simply unable to stay on the bike and suffered numerous falls. He wrote to his friend Faisst: 'Being a beginner, I have so far only learnt to know the dark side of bicycle riding. My poor body is tattooed from bruises I have got in the driving lessons. However, I will continue facing the divine pleasure which is waiting on me ...' [Walker, 1968; Werba, 1971]. Earlier, namely in August 1896, further important evidence can be found in Wolf's medical history. After a train trip to Graz, Wolf was seen by an ophthalmologist for a conjunctival irritation which had been caused by a soot particle. Dr. Elschnigg diagnosed Argyll-Robertson pupils and informed Wolf's friend Heinrich Potpeschnigg, a dentist, about his observation. Wolf, however, was not informed about this finding and its implications [Walker, 1968; Werba, 1971].

September 1897 was the decisive point in Wolf's illness with the overt outbreak of general paresis. His friend Haberlandt was sent a sheet of music with Wolf's handwriting saying: 'Piping hot! Straight from the frying-pan! Am beside myself! Sell me up! Am blissful! Raving!' Haberlandt became suspicious of this strange letter and decided to see him at his apartment in the Schwindgasse. Wolf appeared quite deranged and spoke excitedly about his new opera 'Manuel Venegas'. He sat down at the piano and played and sang from the fragmentary opera in a highly exalted mood, claiming that he had never composed anything so beautiful before. This performance, however, seemed to calm down his spirits and Haberlandt left his friends without anxiety; but Wolf continued composing, 'raging like a volcano', and invited all of his friends on the following Sunday in order to 'play the opera at Perchtoldsdorf to all the faithful'. This date was again preceded by strange letters such as the one to Melanie Köchert, where he urged Melanie to join the audience for his performance: 'If on the same day you don't put in an appearance I shall never again set a foot in your house' [Grasberger, 1991]. The following Saturday September 19, 1897, marked the onset of madness and megalomania. He met his friend Edmund Hellmer for lunch. While eating unusually fast, he picked up the chop he had ordered and simply tore the meat away from the bone, gulping it down like an animal. Suddenly he whispered to Hellmer: 'Did you already know – I have been named director of the Court Opera?' Hellmer first believed Wolf was joking, but Wolf repeated the 'news' when Föll, another friend, arrived. The two friends finally were given a private concert in Wolf's apartment, then Wolf drank brotherhood with them and ended up talking about matters that under normal circumstances he would never have discussed openly – his family, his poverty and his relations with women [Walker, 1968]. The following day, Wolf ran through the streets of Vienna in order to find the singer Hermann

Winkelmann in his duty as the new director of the opera. He aimed at engaging the singer for the same day's concert in Bokmayer's house. Everybody met there at 5 p.m. and Wolf planned to play very recently composed material from his new opera 'Manuel Venegas' on the piano. He started doing so, then tried to play Wagner's prelude to the Meistersinger, but had to interrupt because he could not recall the score by heart. Thereafter, he proclaimed to the audience his nomination as the new director of the Vienna Hofoper and that his first legal act would be dismissing Mahler from his post. Haberlandt had asked Dr. Gorhan from the local hospital to attend the concert as a precaution. Dr. Gorhan diagnosed the outbreak of madness and suggested bringing Wolf to an asylum immediately. The private asylum of Dr. Svetlin in Vienna offered to take Wolf as an inpatient the next morning. Hence, Wolf had to be accompanied back to his home by some friends, where he furiously attacked the housekeeper. His friends had great difficulties to bring this unpleasant scene to an end. On September 21, Wolf was admitted to Dr. Svetlin's asylum – a carriage was sent and Wolf was told that this carriage was bringing him to the opera for the signature of his new contract [Walker, 1968; Werba, 1971; Decsey, 1903–1906; Dorschel, 1985; Hanolka, 1988; Newman, 1966].

A visit Wolf had paid just a short time before to his former roommate and friend from the days in the Vienna conservatory, Gustav Mahler, who had already begun working as the provisional director of the opera, preceded this catastrophe. Both composers had disputed about the plans to produce Wolf's opera 'The Corregidor' at the Vienna court opera which Mahler had previously promised to produce. During the dispute, Mahler finally expressed doubt as to whether the opera would be performed in Vienna at all. Wolf left Mahler raging bitterly and vowing revenge for this disappointment. In this extreme emotional state, Wolf produced the idea that removing the obstacle 'Mahler' would lead the way to his so long merited success, his becoming director of the opera.

Hugo Wolf was discharged in late January 1898 after 4 months in Dr. Svetlin's asylum. His symptoms had improved to a certain degree. For most of the subsequent months his friends would take him on several short holiday trips. This was also the case in October 1898 when the disease broke out again.

During a stay in Traunkirchen Wolf left his apartment one morning tormented by ideas of persecution. His friends searched the vicinity for some time and he was found at the edge of a nearby forest, dripping wet. He had tried to drown himself in the Traunsee, but had finally swum to shore. Then he had wandered in the woods ashamed of what he had attempted to do. He himself asked to be put in a mental home, 'only for god's sake not Svetlin's'. Hence, he was brought to the 'Niederösterreichische Landesirrenanstalt' in Vienna, where he stayed until his death in February 1903 [Walker, 1968; Werba, 1971; Decsey, 1903–1906; Dorschel, 1985; Hanolka, 1988; Newman, 1966].

Similarly in Schumann's case, according to several sources the idea of entering a mental institution was his own. Following a note in his diary on February 10, 1854, a series of auditory delusions occurred. They continued for the following weeks – usually in the form of music. His final piano composition, the 'Ghost variations', was composed as a result of these. Schumann believed the theme to these variations was sent to him by an angel. The hallucinations became more and more horrendous, at times Schumann felt attacked by wild beasts.

At the same time he was obviously afraid of loosing control of his actions and feared harming either himself or someone else. Clara Schumann wrote in her diary that during the night of February 26, Schumann 'suddenly got up and wanted to have his clothes. It was necessary, he said, for him to go into the asylum because he was no longer in control of himself, and did not know what he might do [...] Robert laid out with plain deliberation everything that he wanted to take with him: watch, money, music paper, pens, cigars; and when I said to him: "Robert, do you want to leave your wife and children?", he replied, "it will not be for long. I will soon return cured"' [von Wasielewski,1906].

On the following day, in the midst of the Rhenish carnival in Düsseldorf, Schumann left the house and attempted to take his own life by leaping into the Rhine. In the days that followed, he said to his doctors that 'they should take him to an asylum, because only there could he return to health'. As his treating physician Dr. Richard Hasenclever was acquainted with Dr. Franz Richarz, who owned and led a private asylum in Endenich near Bonn, it was decided to send him there. Schumann arrived in Endenich on March 4 accompanied by Hasenclever and two attendants. At that time it took eight hours to travel from Düsseldorf to Bonn-Endenich. The asylum in Endenich had a good reputation and by all accounts was well maintained [Franken, 1984; Ostwald, 1985].

The recent publication of Robert Schumann's patient records from the Endenich asylum 150 years after his death is important for the understanding of his complex pathography [Franken, 1997a, b; Mayeda et al., 2006]. Due to doctor–patient confidentiality, Dr. Franz Richarz never intended to publish the record; his daughter-in-law bequeathed the record to her godson, a psychiatrist, who was the uncle of Aribert Reimann, a well-known contemporary German composer. Irritated by the fierce and unfair discussion regarding Schumann's final disease, Reimann decided to allow publication of the record [Franken, 1997a, b; Mayeda et al., 2006]. This is a much welcome and most important contribution to a clearer picture of Schumann's final years. In the view of most authors who have since analyzed the material, the diagnosis of neurosyphilis becomes more plausible than it had already been. However, curiously enough, the original sources published by the Schumann Society in Düsseldorf contain the detailed comments of a psychiatrist who makes every attempt to reject this diagnosis [Mayeda et al.,

2006]. Thereby, he stands in a long tradition of authors who favor different disease theories, obviously trying not to tarnish the reputation of the composer and his family [Gruhle, 1906; Kerner, 1963; Möbius, 1906; Nussbaum, 1923; Payk, 1977; Slater and Meyer, 1959]. The given respect may have its origins in the attitude of Clara Schumann, their children and the much protective close friends Johannes Brahms and Joseph Joachim. However, the finally published sources give a very clear picture of neurosyphilis. The following excerpts aim at illustrating the most remarkable symptoms of Schumann's disease.

April 11, 1854: Said to the attendant, the authorities had ordered him to be burnt in hell: he had done too many bad things. During the night very restless, most time out of bed, not taking off the clothes, […] moaned as if in pain, was totally sleepless.

April 19, 1854: Restless at night, spoke loudly to himself until midnight, about the Veneris, being unhappy, becoming mad; got up later and wanted to leave the room, became violent with the attendant.

September 27, 1854: Yesterday moved to the main building: very pleased and thankful thereabout, helping with the transfer … wrote a moderately long, thoughtful and calmly written letter to his wife, with omissions of some words, the date correct. Talked a lot to himself during the night, softly, the fingers moving on the blanket as if playing the piano. Asking the attendant if he had made bad things, somebody mentioned this to him.

November 10, 1854: Almost continuously plays dominos.

December 31, 1854: Rejected sherry and some of the Rhine wine, saying this tasted bitter, similar to the water …

January 8, 1855: … Talking of poison when taking his medication … is so disorganized that becomes impossible for him to have a short communication about a certain object …

January 12, 1855: Was visited by Mr. Brahms yesterday, was very pleased about this visit … talks during the rounds quite freely and understandable but very slowly and with a voice similar to a child (with omissions).

January 22, 1855: … During the rounds reports a spell that made him believe he would die. Said he had never had something similar before, these had been cramps, namely in his right hand … during the rounds – half an hour after the spell – … had convulsions in the fingers and could not suppress them.

January 24, 1855: … Convulsions in the right hand.

February 9, 1855: … Speaks again today about silly things, that the silly voices were calling him.

February 24, 1855: Yesterday in a good mood, talking a lot. Was visited by Mr. Brahms, found him much better than the last time.

March 7, 1855: … The deprivation of sleep being his worst problem, hearing silly voices, a bad demon menacing him, the same having played a lot of horrible animal faces seven months ago, etc.

March 9, 1855: Most of the time his speech is totally incomprehensive.

March 12, 1855: During the rounds sitting on the sofa, a spell of anxiousness with convulsions in his extremities. Complains of headache, pressure in the chest, anxious. The speech very disabled, soundless, unintelligible, afraid of becoming mad. Believes he is persecuted by the Nemesis. His consciousness not disturbed meanwhile … the right pupil is much larger than the left pupil when shining light in his eyes. Understood and answered all questions during the spell.

April 28, 1855: He refers the simplest things to the persecutions of the evil demon. Speaks a lot during visits, but hardly understandable. He expresses the completely unwarranted suspicion that his watch might run too fast.

May 4, 1855: During the rounds writing, unpleasant, said he wrote a letter to a notary in order to sue the doctor.

May 6, 1855: … Today he spoke of the prosecution of the 'wicked hag'. …

May 8, 1855: … Played the piano almost for 2 hours, very wild and incoherent … threatened the attendant with a chair … his speech is mumbling similar to a drunken man.

May 19, 1855: Yesterday very shy, especially after a visit from Joachim, could stay at the piano only for a short period of time, often his whole body was overtaken by shivers and strong convulsions …

May 24, 1855: Played the piano, did not finish the piece, and said this was too tiresome.

June 16, 1855: … Is completely calm, without any symptoms of madness or hallucinations

July 9, 1855: … Says he has pain in his belly, he has pain everywhere on touching him, if he liked.

July 25, 1855: Was agitated, impulsive, loud, struck the attendant, everything being poisoned, during nighttime continuously excited, screaming, angry.

August 25, 1855: Yesterday calm, friendly, talking to himself in an exalted good mood, laughing a lot.

September 8, 1855: … Sometimes very loud today. Could not be persuaded to write a letter to his wife …

September 12, 1855: Wrote down abrupt mentions of melancholic content during the past days and reflections such as: '1831 I was syphilitic and was cured with arsenic'.

October 10, 1855: Since yesterday extremely loud, screaming, shouting, also at night: walks around the room, touching several of his works while shouting: this is mine. Appearance very disordered. […] Poured the wine in the closet, claiming this was urine.

October 31, 1855: Yesterday afternoon, during the whole night and today until after breakfast extremely loud, screaming, consequently very hoarse.

January 19, 1856: During the evening rounds friendly, tried to talk coherently and calmly about his compositions.

April 16, 1856: Was calm, burned the letters from his wife yesterday evening and this morning … disagrees that he burned letters at all ...

April 29, 1856: Yesterday wrote a clear and coherent letter to his doctors …

June 9, 1856: Yesterday received birthday greeting from Mr. Brahms; was unpleasant, speaking of poison when hot chocolate was served.

July 11, 1856: … looking sick. His eyes squinting inside. His pupils both much widened.

Final Illness and Death

Franz Schubert

Schubert's final disease began on October 31, 1828, when he left a fish dinner full of disgust. However, on November 3, he was able to walk to the church

---

in Hernals, a three-hour walk [Hetenyi, 1986; Deutsch, 1921/1922]. There is a strange anecdote just before Schubert fell seriously ill, he appeared accompanied by Josef Lanz at Simon Sechter's house in order to start special lessons on fugues. The well-known master of musical theory gave a first lesson to his new scholars, but for the second lesson only Lanz reappeared informing Sechter that Schubert was seriously ill. In his last letter of November 12, 1828, Schubert wrote to Schober: 'Dear Schober, I am ill. I have eaten nothing for eleven days and have drunk nothing. I totter feebly and shakily from my chair to bed and back again. Rinna is treating me; if I ever take anything, I bring it up at once' [Deutsch, 1964]. Until that day, he had been working on an opera and correcting the proofs of his song cycle 'Die Winterreise'.

Schubert's brother Ferdinand recorded the finances needed for his brother's treatment: one can find expenses for blood-letting on November 13, medicines, ointments and powders (on one occasion more specifically mustard powder) and vesicant plasters which would have contained the blistering agent cantharidin [Deutsch, 1921/1922]. When Dr. Rinna von Sarenbach fell sick, he was replaced by his friend Dr. Josef von Vering. Whether or not by chance, von Vering was a famous specialist in the treatment of syphilis, having published two well-known books on this topic. He had no hope of saving Schubert's life due to 'advanced disintegration of the blood'. Together with his colleague Dr. Johann Baptist Wisgrill, whom he brought in for a consultation, they diagnosed 'Nervenfieber' (nervous fever) and ordered a second male nurse in addition to the female nurse because Schubert's care was becoming increasingly complex [Deutsch, 1921/1922]. His symptoms worsened and he became delirious, tried to escape from bed and had to be restrained. On November 18, he hallucinated, imagined that he was in a strange room, and asked his brother to take him to his own room. Obviously, he thought he was being buried alive and felt himself close to Beethoven's grave. Schubert died in the afternoon of November 19, 1828.

There are several details arguing against the most often cited diagnosis of typhoid fever as Schubert's final illness. At least, the diagnosis of Nervenfieber by the treating physicians was definitely not used as a synonym for typhoid fever at that time [Hetenyi, 1986]. Nervenfieber is a very nonspecific term referring to a concurrence of fever and cerebral symptoms. On the other hand, Schubert's Nervenfieber may well have been a symptom of meningovascular syphilis occurring on average 7 years after the primary syphilis infection. Therefore, we can understand Schubert's prodromal symptoms of headaches, vertigo and intermittent focal symptoms, aphonia and inability to play the piano for a while, and also the final therapeutics including ointments and vesicant plasters. On the other hand, whether mercury poisoning played an important role, as suggested by some authors, remains speculative.

Robert Schumann

The final entrances in Robert Schumann's record from Endenich read as follows:

July 29, 1856: Calm from noon on, at night as well, taking some teaspoons of wine jelly and some wine from his wife …
July 30, 1856: Yesterday at 1 o'clock in the afternoon 60 breaths, pulse almost not intelligible. Died yesterday at 4 p.m. Begin autopsy on July 30, at 3:30 p.m.

Clara reports: 'He suffered terribly, although the doctor said differently. His limbs were in continual convulsions. His speaking was often very vehement. Ah! I prayed to God to release him, because I loved him so'. Schumann died in his sleep on July 29, at 4 p.m. Clara saw him a half hour later: 'I stood by the corpse of my dearly beloved husband and was at peace; all my feelings went in thanks to God that he was finally free' [von Wasielewski, 1906].

Hugo Wolf

Also Hugo Wolf seemingly died in a moment when, besides his attendant, none of his friends, who had waited at his deathbed for many days, were with him. Pneumonia was considered the final illness, high fever and horrible seizures are reported from his last visitors. Wolf is buried in the Central Cemetery in Vienna, along with many other notable composers [Walker, 1968; Werba, 1971].

Synopsis of Symptoms and Disease Course in Schumann and Wolf

According to the seminal works of Franken [1997a, b, 1984], the disease courses of both Schumann and Wolf are so similar that one can hardly diagnose separate illnesses. A series of cardinal symptoms of general paresis can be derived from the sources (table 1). The latency between the infection and the outbreak of general paresis was 22 years in Schumann and 20 years in Wolf. This was preceded by a neurasthenic prodromal phase in both, although part of the 'neurasthenic' behavior may have been a result of marked personality traits. Wolf died 5 years after the onset of general paresis, Schumann survived for 30 months. Hallucinations with acoustic, visual, and scenic content were present in both. Paranoid features such as the fear of being poisoned are found in Schumann's patient records on several occasions and are reported in Hugo Wolf's as well. The latter also displayed delusions of grandeur, at times he would claim to be Jupiter and control the weather. Once he wrote to his friends: 'It would be my plan to go on worldwide tours with the Weimar theatrical personnel, much as the Meiningen troupe did, who in their time cre-

Table 1. Symptoms and disease course of Robert Schumann and Hugo Wolf

Symptoms	Schumann	Wolf
Latency between infection and outbreak of general paresis	22 years	20 years
Neurasthenic prodromal phase	Present	Present
Latency between outbreak of general paresis and death	2.5–3 years	5.5 years
Hallucinations and paranoia	Marked without delusions of grandeur	Marked with delusions of grandeur
Aggressive behavior	Often and markedly expressed	Often and markedly expressed
Focal and generalized seizures	Present	Present
Dysarthria	Present, progressing to anarthria	Present, progressing to anarthria
Pupillary disturbances	Pupils of different size, strabism	Argyll-Robertson pupils
Stereotypies	Marked	Present
Fear of being poisoned	Permanent	At times
Cachexia, incontinence	Marked at final stage	Marked at final stage
Pneumonia as final event	Present	Present
Personality change	Present	Present
Loss of writing ability	Not before 1856	After 1899
Gave up composing	After 1854	After 1899

Modified, according to Franken [1997a].

ated a great and justified sensation. But the project I have in mind would have an infinitely greater appeal to the public, as works of mine (and exclusively mine) would be performed, which are never to appear in print; therefore they could not be conveyed to the public in any other way than under my direction'. Aggressive behavior was present in both composers as well as focal seizures. Generalized seizures were also reported during their final days, along with pneumonia as the terminal illness. Already some time before marked cachexia was noted, incontinence was documented. Dysarthria was a very important and marked symptom in both composers, and pupillary abnormalities were observed by medical doctors before the onset of general paresis in Wolf's case and in Schumann's record from Endenich. Schumann showed marked stereotypies in playing dominos for whole days. From a visit in Endenich, Brahms reported finding Schumann with an atlas, arranging names of cities and rivers in alphabetical order: 'We sat down, it became increasingly pain-ful for me [...] He spoke continually, but I understood nothing [...] Often he only babbled, something like babab-dadada […]'. Schumann permanently feared of being poisoned, and would therefore often refuse his food. On other occasions he poured wine on the floor claiming it was urine. Both composer's writing ability deteriorated. Wolf's handwriting became unintelligible from 1899 on. A late document of his signature from 1899 shows significantly disabled handwriting. Robert Schumann, in contrast, could write quite well until a year before he died. His last letter to Clara shows clear handwriting with only minor semantic errors. Regarding the creative output, both composers did not manage to compose new oeuvres. Schumann's 'Geistervariationen' is probably his final original work; although in the early days at Endenich it is reported that Schumann composed a piano accompaniment to a Paganini piece for violin and two short and very simple chorale settings (the first on the church chorale 'when my last hour is close at hand') which have been published posthumously.

Syphilis and Lied Composition – Two Sides of a Medal

In an interview about a Hugo Wolf program at the 2003 Salzburg Festival, the famous singer Thomas Hampson compared the composer's work rhythms to a 'light bulb that is about to go out but, before that happens, gives off an especially bright, hot light for one last time' [http://www.hampsong.com/blog/images/uploads/Salzburg_Aug04_2003_O.pdf]. Hampson assumes that this was surely related to his disease and speaks of the same phenomenon in the work of Franz Schubert and Robert Schumann, all of them known as the three most important German composers of Lieder who suffered from syphilis. In all three composers, periods of 'a frenzy of creativity' were followed by 'sudden fading' [http://www.hampsong.com/blog/images/uploads/Salzburg_Aug04_2003_O.pdf]. He finally asks the questions whether the 'illness released in them a heightened sensibility for lyric form, emotional surges, and sensitivity that empowered them to achieve such masterly settings?' And furthermore: 'Would they have produced Lieder in such quantities if they hadn't been infected?'. It is certainly very reassuring for the medical pathographer to also have an artist asking these most important and interesting questions.

Definitely the clusters of productivity in Schubert, Schumann and Wolf are most amazing. Series of Lied compositions were produced in the shortest periods of time. This is even more remarkable when looking at the total number of songs in their complete oeuvre and the relatively short periods of productive life.

The 'heightened sensibility for lyric form' was probably very well nourished in the romantic era. At a first glance, the personalities of the two composers, however, do not seem to have been susceptible to the 'exaggerated' emotional states of romanticism. From our point of view, the composers' social competence was not perfect in any sense – for instance Wasielewsky reported that Schumann 'lacked the ability to put himself in close rapport with others, and to make his meaning clear to them; this was because he either was silent or spoke so low that he could not be understood' [von Wasielewski, 1906]. Yet, both had definite strengths in expressing their points of view in the written word. Possibly their way to overcome these personal 'shortcomings' was to concentrate on musical expression as a way of showing emotions.

The role of illness is in part quite obvious. All three composers may well have been suspicious about the nature of the primary infection – the medical knowledge of contemporary physicians was good enough to indicate to their patients the possible serious consequences of their sexual adventures. Hence, it may well have been more than the 'typical' anxiety of the period that both Schumann and Wolf expressed their fear of becoming mad. In addition, they were very well aware of the fates of their famous 'co-patients'. Ironically, in a megalomanic delusion Wolf expressed his ambitions to cure Nietzsche and was convinced that he was the director of his asylum in Vienna. Schumann and Wolf must have had in mind the horrible vision of ending in an asylum; they were by all accounts well aware of the shortness of their remaining productive time. By all means, this alone, would have justified an intense concentration and condensation of their respective productive periods.

The less obvious role of their illness lies in the potential catalytic effect of the disease with respect to creativity. This is by far the more difficult question to answer. Several authors have speculated about the nature of the very wide mood swings and have proposed the diagnosis of bipolar affective disorder in both composers to explain the marked mood swings and also fitting with periods of feverish creativity.

However, even allowing for such a diagnosis, it certainly does not explain the final period of illnesses. Again, syphilis alone is definitely not a sufficient diagnosis to explain all of the remarkable extremes in creative output in Schubert, Schumann and Wolf. Whatever Schubert died of, it did not affect his genius. In clear contrast, in both Schumann and Wolf neurosyphilis was the due cause of the final termination in artistic output. Hence, we can only speculate about the possible link between neurosyphilis and creativity through the severe organic disturbance of the neuronal networks including the limbic brain with its direct links to motivation. Likewise, a disease-mediated disinhibition of the frontal-subcortical circuits might interfere with creativity.

References

Böhme G: Medizinische Porträts berühmter Komponisten, Band 2. Stuttgart, Fischer, 1987.

Boucourechliev A: Robert Schumann. Reinbek bei Hamburg, Rowohlt, 1958.

Decsey E: Hugo Wolf. Leipzig, Schuster u. Löffler, 1903–1906.

Deutsch OE: Schuberts Krankheit. Z Musikwissenschaft 1921/1922;4:100–106.

Deutsch OE: Schubert. Die Erinnerungen seiner Freunde. Leipzig, VEB Breitkopf und Härtel, 1957.

Deutsch OE: Schubert. Die Dokumente seines Lebens. Kassel, Bärenreiter, 1964.

Dorschel A: Hugo Wolf. Reinbek bei Hamburg, Rowohlt, 1985.

Eismann G, Nauhaus G (eds): Schumann R: Tagebücher, 3 Vols. Leipzig, Deutscher Verlag für Musik, 1971–1987.

Franken FH: Untersuchungen zur Krankengeschichte Schumanns; in Robert-Schumann-Gesellschaft Düsseldorf (eds): Robert Schumann – Ein romantisches Erbe in neuer Forschung. Mainz, Schott, 1984.

Franken FH: Franz Schubert; in: Die Krankheiten grosser Komponisten, Band 2. Wilhelmshafen, Noetzel, 1989.

Franken FH: Die Krankheiten grosser Komponisten, Vol. 4. Wilhelmshafen, Noetzel, 1997a.

Franken FH: Robert Schumann in der Irrenanstalt Endenich. Zum aufgefundenen ärztlichen Verlaufsbericht 1854–1856 von Doktor Franz Richarz; in: Brahms Studien, Band 11. Tutzing, Hans Schneider, 1997b.

Grasberger F: Hugo Wolf: Letters to Melanie Köchert. Translated by Louise McClelland Urban. New York, Schirmer Books, 1991.

Gruhle HW: Brief über Robert Schumann's Krankheit an P.J. Möbius. Zbl Nervenheilk Psychiatrie 1906;26:805–810.

Hanolka K: Hugo Wolf: Sein Leben, sein Werk, seine Zeit. Stuttgart, Deutsche Verlags-Anstalt, 1988.

Hellmer E: Hugo Wolf: Erlebtes und Erlauschtes. Wien, Wiener Literarische Anstalt, 1921.

Hernried R: Hugo Wolf's Corregidor at Mannheim. Musical Quarterly 1940;26:19–30.

Hernried R: Hugo Wolf's 'four operas': with unpublished letters by Hugo Wolf, Rosa Mayreder, and Oskar Grohe. Musical Quarterly 1945;31:89–100.

Hetenyi G: The terminal illness of Franz Schubert and the treatment of syphilis in Vienna in the eighteen hundred and twenties. Can Bull Med Hist 1986;3:51–65.

Hopkins Porter C: The reign of the 'Dilettanti': Dusseldorf from Mendelssohn to Schumann Musical Quarterly 1989;73:476–512.

Kerner D: Krankheiten grosser Musiker, Stuttgart, Schattauer, 1963.

Kerner D, Schadewald E: Grosse Musiker. Leben und Leiden, 5. Aufl. Stuttgart, Schattauer, 1998.

Mahler A: Gustav Mahler: Erinnerungen und Briefe. Amsterdam, A. de Lange, 1940.

Mayeda A, Niemöller KW, Appel BR (eds): Robert Schumann in Endenich (1854–1856): Krankenakten, Briefzeugnisse und zeitgenössische Berichte. Mainz, Schott, 2006.

Möbius PJ: Über Robert Schumanns Krankheit. Halle, Marhold, 1906.

Newbould B: Schubert. The Music and the Man. Berkeley, University of California Press, 1999.

Newman E: Hugo Wolf. New York, Dover Publications, 1966.

Neyses J: Robert Schumann als Musikdirektor in Düsseldorf. Düsseldorfer Almanach 1927;71:73–74.

Nussbaum F: Der Streit über Schumanns Krankheit; Diss. Köln, 1923.

Ostwald P: Schumann. The Inner Voices of a Musical Genius. Boston, Northeastern University Press, 1985.

Payk TR: Robert Schumann als Patient in Bonn-Endenich. Confin Psychiatr 1977;20;153–161.

Sams E: Schubert's illness re-examined. Musical Times 1980;131:15–22.

Schirlbauer A: Das zeitgenössische Ölporträt Schuberts hat seinen Maler gefunden: Anton Depauly. Neues zu dem einst Mähler, Ebyl oder Kupelwieser zugeschriebenen Schubert-Gemälde in der Portrait-Galerie der Gesellschaft der Musikfreunde in Wien, Schubert: Perspektiven, 4 (2004), 145–173.

Singh AE, Romanowski B: Syphilis: review with emphasis on clinical, epidemiologic, and some biologic features. Clin Microbiol Rev 1999;12:187–209.

Slater E, Meyer A: Contributions to a pathography of the musicians: 1. Robert Schumann. Confin Psychiatr 1959;2:65–94.

Solomon M: Franz Schubert and the Peacocks of Benvenuto Cellini. 19th Century Music 1989;12:193–206.

Walker F: Conversations with Hugo Wolf. Music Lett 1960;41:5–12.

Walker F: Hugo Wolf: A Biography. New York, Knopf, 1968.

Werba E: Hugo Wolf oder der zornige Romantiker. Wien, Molden, 1971.

von Wasielewski WJ: Robert Schumann. Eine Biographie. Dresden, 1858; in Wasielewski D (ed): 4. umgearbeitete und beträchtlich vermehrte Auflage. Leipzig, Breitkopf & Härtel, 1906.

Prof. Dr. Hansjörg Bäzner
Neurologische Klinik, Klinikum Stuttgart, Bürgerhospital
Tunzhofer Strasse 14–16
DE–70191 Stuttgart (Germany)
Tel. +49 711 278 22401, Fax +49 711 278 22174, E-Mail H.Baezner@klinikum-stuttgart.de

Bogousslavsky J, Hennerici MG, Bäzner H, Bassetti C (eds): Neurological Disorders in Famous
Artists – Part 3. Front Neurol Neurosci. Basel, Karger, 2010, vol 27, pp 84–91

....

Hector Berlioz and Other Famous Artists with Opium Abuse

Paul L. Wolf

Department of Pathology, Veterans Administration Health Science Medical Center,
University of California at San Diego, Director of Autopsy, Hematology and
Coagulation Laboratory, Veterans Administration Medical Center,
San Diego, Calif., USA

Abstract

The effect of opium on the creativity and productivity of a famous composer of classical music, an essayist, and poets including Hector Berlioz, Thomas De Quincy, Samuel Taylor Coleridge, John Keats, and Jean Cocteau, is described. Opium is a narcotic drug prepared from the juice of the unripe seed capsules of the opium poppy. It contains alkaloids such as morphine, codeine, and papaverine. Medically it is used to relieve pain and produce sleep. It is used as an intoxicant. Alcohol and opium were commonly relied on in the 19th century, especially by artists, to stimulate creativity and relieve stress. These artists described the effect of opium on their creativity and productivity.

The effect of opium on the creativity and productivity of a famous composer of classical music, an essayist, and poets is described. Opium is a narcotic drug prepared from the juice of the unripe seed capsules of the opium poppy. It contains alkaloids such as morphine, codeine, and papaverine. Opium has been utilized to relieve pain and as a soporific. It is also considered to be an intoxicant. Opium was used by artists in the 19th century to stimulate creativity and relieve pain and stress. The artists described the influence of opium on their creativity and productivity [Wolf, 2005].

Hector Berlioz (1803–1869; fig. 1) was known for his orchestrating genius, his long interrupted melodies and his way of relating his musical compositions to stories and ideas. Hector Berlioz was one of the best composers of classical music in France. One of his most famous creations was 'Symphonie

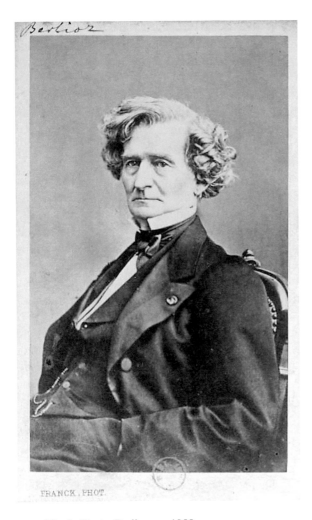

Fig. 1. Hector Berlioz, ca. 1855.

Fantastique'. His other notable pieces were: 'Harold in Italy, a Symphony'; 'Roméo and Juliet, a Symphony'; 'Roman Carnival Overture'; 'The Damnation of Faust, an Orchestral Cantata'; 'Béatrice et Bénédict, an Opera'; 'Benvenuto Cellini, an Opera', and 'Les Trojans, an Opera'.

Berlioz's father was a physician, who attempted to interest his son in becoming a physician. His father also taught him to appreciate classical literature and classical music. His father provided Berlioz with a flute, a guitar and piano lessons. Berlioz was also admired as a classical music conductor, critic, and writer. His books on music include 'The Treatise on Modern Instrumentation' and 'Orchestration and Evenings with the Orchestra' and two volumes of 'Memoirs'. Berlioz first enrolled in a medical school in Paris. However, after his first year, he gave up medicine and became a music student at the Paris Conservatory of Music. Berlioz had severely carious teeth and agonizing toothaches for which he medicated himself with opium to relieve the pain. This was thus the cause for his overuse of opium [Wolf, 2005].

As a boy, Berlioz adored both music and literature, and he went on to compose the 'Symphonie Fantastique', in which the hero (a thinly disguised representation of Berlioz himself) supposedly survives a large dose of narcotic. Another interpretation of the 'Symphonie Fantastique' is that it describes the dreams of a jilted lover (Berlioz), possibly attempting suicide by an overdose of opium. This work is a milestone marking the beginning of the Romantic era of music. His creativity was enhanced in particular by a love of great literature and an unquenchable passion of the feminine ideal, and in the best of his works these elements conspired to produce music of exquisite beauty.

Berlioz took opium to relieve agonizing toothaches, but there is no indication that he ever took opium to become intoxicated, as the author Thomas De Quincy did. On September 11, 1827, Berlioz attended a performance of 'Hamlet' at the Paris Odeon, in which the actress Harriet Smithson (Berlioz later called her Ophelia and Henrietta) played the role of Ophelia. Overwhelmed by her beauty and charismatic stage presence, he fell desperately in love. The grim program of 'Symphonie Fantastique' was born out of Berlioz's despair due to the unrequited love he had for the Shakespearean actress Harriet Smithson.

Berlioz found a way to channel his emotional upheaval, of 'I'Affaire Smithson' into something he could control, that is, a 'fantastic symphony' that took as its subject the experiences of a young musician in love. A detailed program Berlioz wrote prior to a performance of the 'Symphonie Fantastique', and which he later revised, leaves no doubt that he conceived this symphony as a romantically heightened self-portrait. Berlioz did eventually woo and win Miss Smithson, and they were married in 1833 at the British Embassy in Paris. The program Berlioz wrote for 'Symphonie Fantastique' reads, in part: 'A young musician of morbid sensibility and ardent imagination in a paroxysm of love-sick despair has poisoned himself with opium. The drug, too weak to kill, plunges him into a heavy sleep accompanied by strange visions. His sensations, feelings, and memories are translated in his sick brain into musical images and ideas' [Goulding, 1992].

Berlioz's program for each of the five movements are as follows.

First Movement: Dreams and Passions

Berlioz recalls an uneasiness of his soul with melancholy and joy which he experienced before seeing Ms. Smithson whom he loves, followed by immense love with which she inspired in him.

Second Movement: The Ball

Berlioz sees Ms. Smithson at a ball in the midst of a tumult of a brilliant fete.

Third Movement: Scenes in the Country

Early in the movement, the music is tranquil, until Ms. Smithson appears causing his heart to stop beating and he becomes agitated fearing that she will reject him.

Fourth Movement: The March to the Gallows

Berlioz dreams that he has killed his beloved and he is condemned to death and led to execution.

Fifth Movement: Dreams of the Witches' Sabbath

Berlioz sees himself at a witches' Sabbath in the midst of a group of ghosts and monsters. A grotesque dance occurs. Ms. Smithson appears and howls, as joy takes place at her arrival [Cross and Ewen, 1962].

Berlioz eventually married Ms. Smithson. However, she turned out to be a shrew and an alcoholic, and they eventually separated.

The underlying 'theme' of the 'Symphonie Fantastique' is obsessive with unfulfilled love. The symphony reflects Berlioz's hysteric nature with fits of frenzy, as revealed in his dramatic behavior in conducting a symphony (fig. 2). It was obvious that Berlioz was addicted to opium, which is a yellow to dark brown addictive narcotic drug prepared from the juice of the unripe seed capsules of the opium poppy. It contains alkaloids such as morphine, codeine, and papaverine, and is used as an intoxicant. Medically, it is used to relieve pain and produce sleep. It is a tranquilizer and has a stupefying effect. Apart from alcohol, opium was the drug most commonly relied on in the 19th century, especially by artists to stimulate creative ability and relieve stress. An overdose of opium may cause death due to respiratory failure. Nonfatal signs and symptoms include restlessness, agitation, and convulsions [Dreisbach, 1983].

Berlioz's marriage to Ms. Smithson was not a happy one. Both were extremely temperamental. Ms. Smithson suffered from the anguishes of an excellent actress whose star had been eclipsed. She became ill and an invalid and died. A year later he remarried a singer named Marie Recio.

Berlioz continued to be creative and productive composing 'Harold in Italy', 'The Requiem', 'Roméo and Juliet', 'The Damnation of Faust', 'TeDeum', 'Enfance du Christ', and the operas, 'Benvenuto Cellini', 'Les Trojans', and 'Béatrice et Bénédict'. He also composed many choral works and songs. His financial status as a composer was not good which caused him to turn to music criticism. He was considered to be the best critic of his time. He also turned to

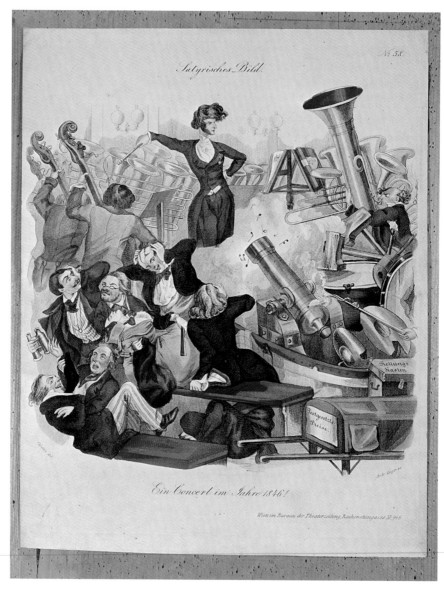

Fig. 2. Hector Berlioz conducting one of his symphonies. Satirical print depicting listeners fleeing the noise. Located at the Historisches Museum der Stadt Wien, Vienna, Austria. Eric Lessing, Art Resource, New York, N.Y., reprinted with permission.

conducting in his later years. Within a few years, he became dejected and died in 1869. Opium certainly influenced the creativity and productivity of Hector Berlioz's musical career, especially in his 'Symphonie Fantastique'. The last few years of Berlioz's life were unhappy. His productive years were over, he became ill, and his second marriage failed [Schonberg, 1981].

Thomas De Quincey (1785–1859) was an English essayist. He wrote a rare kind of imaginative prose that was highly ornate, full of subtle rhythms, and sensitive to the sound and arrangement of words. His prose was as much musical as literary in its style and structure, and he developed such modern narrative techniques as stream-of-consciousness.

De Quincey authored his most famous essay, 'Confessions of an English Opium-Eater', in 1821. He authored an eloquent essay on both the delights and the agonies of opium abuse. He believed that the habit of using opium was of common practice in is day and was not considered a vice. Originally, De Quincey believed that the use of opium was not to seek pleasure, but intended for his extreme facial pain which was caused by trigeminal neuralgia. The essay's biographical parts are important mainly as background to the dreams De Quincey described later. In these dreams, he examined (with the help of opium) the intimate workings of memory and the subconscious. It is easily understandable that De Quincey 'began to use opium as an article of daily diet'. He was addicted to the drug from the age of 19 until he died. The pain was not the only reason for his addiction; he also discovered the effect of opium on his spiritual life. By accident, he met a college acquaintance who recommended opium for his pain. On a rainy Sunday in London, De Quincy visited a druggist's shop, where he asked for a tincture of opium. He arrived at his lodgings and lost not a moment in taking the quantity prescribed. In an hour, he stated: 'Oh heavens! What a revulsion, what a resurrection, from its lowest depths of the inner spirit! What an apocalypse of the world within me! That my pains had vanished was now a trifle in my eyes; this negative effect was swallowed up in the immensity of these positive effects, which had opened before me, in the abyss of divine enjoyment thus suddenly revealed. Here was a panacea for all human woes; here was the secret of happiness, about which philosophers had disputed for so may ages, at once discovered; happiness might now be bought for a penny and carried in the waistcoat-pocket; portable ecstasies might be corked up in a pint-bottle' [Sandblom, 1996].

Other famous writers and poets used opium. Samuel Taylor Coleridge (1772–1834) was the most brilliant English writer of his generation. Coleridge's inability to concentrate and to carry to full potentiality the expression of his genius as a poet was a cause of his acute suffering. The roots of it were in his temperament, aggravated by his long periods of addiction to opium which ruined his health and sapped his vitality.

Coleridge claimed to have composed the 'Kublai Khan' in a dream as a psychological curiosity. He was a pioneer in the discovery and exploitation of the unconscious and this poem looks forward to later symbolism and surrealism. Coleridge saw the palace of the Kublai Khan in a trance and sang its praise 'in a state of Reverie, caused by 2 grains of opium'. Coleridge wrote: 'For he on honeydew hath fed/And drunk the milk of Paradise'. John Keats (1795–1821) was the most remarkable of the English Romantic poets. The output of this great poet was very productive in his life of 24 years. He wrote, 'I find I cannot exist without poetry'. Early, he trained in a surgical medical practice. He abandoned surgical medicine two years later to devote his life to poetry. Keats also tried opium and stated in his 'Ode to Melancholy': 'My heart aches, and a drowsy numbness pains/My sense, as although of hemlock I had drunk/Or emptied some dull opiate to the drains'. He contracted tuberculosis, which was a common fatal illness, and died in February 1821 [Spender and Hall, 1970].

Jean Cocteau (1891–1963) was famous as a novelist and poet. His novel, 'Les Enfants Terribles', about emotionally disturbed adolescents is one of his best-known books. He used opium as an aid to recover mental balance. He wrote, 'I preferred an artificial harmony to no harmony at all'. His self-portrait in a journal, 'D'une Desintoxication', depicts the ordeal of weaning off the cure from opium and how he was helped by creativity. He stated, 'Sweat and bile precede some phantom substance which would have dissolved, leaving no other trace behind except a deep depression. If writing had not given it a direction, relief and shape – after the cure came the worse moment, the worse danger, health with his void and an immense sadness. The doctors hand you over to suicide' [Sandblom, 1996].

The effect of opium on a famous composer of classical music, an essayist, and poets is analyzed here, including their use of opium, their illnesses, and their famous artistic works. The association between the use of opium, illness, and art may be close [Osler, 1920]. Although they were intoxicated with opium and suffered from various illnesses, they continued to be productive [Weatherall, 1994]. Opium and their illnesses influenced their creativity and productivity [Wolf, 1994].

References

Cross M, Ewen O: Encyclopedia of the Great Composers and Their Music, 2 ed, revised. Garden City, Doubleday, 1962, vol 1.

Dreisbach RH: Handbook of Poisoning, 11 ed. Los Altos, Lance Medical, 1983.

Goulding PG: Classical Music. New York, Fawcett Books, 1992.

Osler W: The Old Humanities and the New Science. Boston, Houghton Mifflin, 1920, pp 26–28.

Sandblom P: Creativity and Disease, 9 ed. New York, Marion Boyers, 1996.

Schonberg HC: The Lives of the Great Composers, 2 ed, revised., New York, Norton, 1981.

Spender S, Hall D: The Concise Encyclopedia of English and American Poets and Poetry, 2 ed, Revised in new format. London, Hutchinson, 1970.

Weatherall D: The inhumanity of medicine. BMJ 1994;309:1671–1672.

Wolf PL: If clinical chemistry had existed then. Clin Chem 1994;40:328–335.

Wolf PL: The effects of diseases, drugs, and chemicals on the creativity and productivity of famous sculptors, classic painters, classic music composers, and authors. Arch Pathol Lab Med 2005; 129: 1457–1464.

Paul L. Wolf, MD
University of California, Medical Center
200 W Arbor Drive
San Diego, CA 92103 (USA)
Tel. +1 858 552 8585/Ext. 7762, Fax +1 858 552 7452, E-Mail paul.wolf@med.va.gov

Bogousslavsky J, Hennerici MG, Bäzner H, Bassetti C (eds): Neurological Disorders in Famous
Artists – Part 3. Front Neurol Neurosci. Basel, Karger, 2010, vol 27, pp 92–100

....

Shostakovich and ALS

Veena R. Kalapatapu, Aedan P. Gilkey, Robert M. Pascuzzi

Department of Neurology, Indiana University School of Medicine, Indiana Clinic,
Clarian Health, Indianapolis, Ind., USA

Abstract

The life of the Russian composer Dmitri Dmitriyevich Shostakovich (25 September
1903 – 9 August 1975) was marked by chronic ill health. There is evidence that he suffered
from a progressive asymmetric weakness of the limbs. The diagnosis of his condition eluded
multiple physicians and was never conclusively identified. Despite enduring an insidious
20-year course, Shostakovich remained a prolific composer and performer. His remarkable
cultural contributions, in the setting of such adversity, continue to inspire other people beset
with chronic paralytic illnesses such as amyotrophic lateral sclerosis.

Copyright © 2010 S. Karger AG, Basel

Dmitri Dmitriyevich Shostakovich was born September 25, 1906. His parents were Dmitri and Sophia Shostakovich. He died at the Kremlin hospital in
August of 1975. He was married to Nina Vasilievna from 1934 until her death
in 1954. She was the mother of Shostakovich's two children, Maxim and Galya.
In 1962 Shostakovich married Irina Antonova, who lives in Moscow and has
been instrumental in the preservation of his legacy.

The works of Dmitri Dmitriyevich Shostakovich, including symphonies,
chamber music, concertos, and a rich treasury of film scores, have enter-
tained and intrigued audiences for over half a century. Many of his compositions reflect the social and political events of Stalin-led Russia, especially
the conflict between government and individual freedom of artistic expression [White, 2008]. Other pieces are simply charming, lyrical, and clever
(such as his music for children). Shostakovich composed the 2nd Piano
Concerto for his son Maxim, who was completing his training in music.
(Maxim Shostakovich has had his own illustrious career as a conductor.)
Listening to the 2nd movement, one can experience the compelling beauty in
Shostakovich's music, and be forever drawn to the man and his art.

After Stalin's death on March 6, 1953, Shostakovich experienced a sense of liberation. On December 17 of the same year, the Leningrad Philharmonic performed the 10th Symphony, which reflected his perceptions of Stalin. It was not until Krushchev became Party Leader in 1956 that Shostakovich began to receive recognition in Soviet Russia and worldwide [Roseberry, 1981]. Sadly, it was about this time that Shostakovich's health was beginning to deteriorate. Though present as early as 1958, signs of his disease were little noticed by the public for some time.

Shostakovich's Neurological Disorder

Shostakovich's early health has been summarized by Elizabeth Wilson in her compelling biography entitled 'Shostakovich – A Life Remembered' [1994]. Quoting from her book:

'Throughout his life, Shostakovich suffered from bad health. His fragile constitution had been undermined in childhood and adolescence by cold and hunger, and by a bout of tuberculosis. With his sensitive, almost neurotic disposition, he tended to react physically to the outward circumstances of his life. Even before the first symptoms of a debilitating illness manifested itself in 1958, the composer spent much time in hospitals and sanitoria for cures and checkups.'

While a number of sources suggest that the chronic debilitating illness (presumably amyotrophic lateral sclerosis, ALS) began in 1958, we speculate that the beginning can be traced to an earlier time. From the DSCH Journal, a piece entitled 'The Last Summer Together' written by Irina Vassilyevna-Varzar (translated for DSCH by Joan Pemberton-Smith) states: '1954 was the last summer that the whole Shostakovich family – Mitya (Shostakovich), my sister Nina, and the children, Galya and Maxim – all spent together' [Varzar, 1994]. In her moving memoir she recalls, in 1954,

'That summer, Mitya used to go on long cycle rides with the children but Maxim used to complain: "Poppa, you're making us slow down – you can't keep up with us!" Mitya worried about the children, so he used to set a time for their return, and put Alla's (my daughter's) watch on his arm, being the most reliable. Once he fell into a ditch and tore his suit … how hard it was to keep up with those young rascals'.

It is possible that this description of his being unable to 'keep up with us' on long cycle rides reflects the earliest symptoms of weakness in the limbs, particularly the legs.

By 1958 Shostakovich had sufficient symptoms to clearly indicate the presence of a neurological disorder. Wilson quotes from a letter that Shostakovich wrote to his friend Isaak Glikman in 1958 [1994]:

'My right hand became very weak. I often have pins and needles. I cannot lift heavy things. My fingers can grip hold of any suitcase, but I cannot hang a coat up on a hook. I find it difficult to brush my teeth. When I write my hand gets tired. I can only play [the piano] slowly and pianissimo. I noticed this condition in Paris where I was barely able to play my concerts. I just took no notice. The high priests of medicine are unable to answer my question as to what name to give this illness; they have condemned me to a stay in a hospital' [Wilson, 1994].

Wilson [1994] chronicles the composer's subsequent physical deterioration as follows:

'In 1960, at his son's Maxim's wedding, his legs suddenly gave away, resulting in the fracture of his left leg. Seven years later he broke his right leg, and remained visibly lame for the rest of his life. With stoic humor he reported from hospital to Glikman: "We're 75% there. My right leg is broken, my left leg is broken, my right hand is damaged. All it needs is for me to hurt my left hand, and then 100% of my extremities will be out of order"' [Wilson, 1994].

'It was only towards the end of 1965 that his condition was successfully diagnosed by the Leningrad doctor D.K. Bogorodinsky, as a form of poliomyelitis which affected the nerve endings and the bones. Shostakovich jokingly referred to his having contracted a "children's disease", but came to resent more and more the humiliation of it being difficult to walk and use his hands' [Wilson, 1994].

Perhaps this portrayal of Shostakovich as nervous and hesitant provides a glimpse of an ailing and fearful man who senses his body failing him.

By this time, Shostakovich had gone through several ups and downs in his career during the era of Stalinism in the Soviet. Around his 60th birthday, Shostakovich was awarded the title Hero of Socialist Labor by the Soviet Union. Though he had received awards from Finland, Rome, and the US, this was the first time Shostakovich was officially recognized by his own country. Unfortunately, by this time, Shostakovich was already feeling despondent. Reporters and journalists stated,

'...wretchedly pallid stare and nervous, twitching fingers; "the inscrutable face with its strange tremor" of a man prone to silent misery or a jabbering spate of words. His doctors had banned cigarettes and alcohol, and the result was a composer's block which it took smuggled brandy to cure' [Jackson, 1997].

Shostakovich wrote to his friend Glikman in 1966:

'During my stay in hospital I was examined by professors Michelson (a surgeon) and Schmidt (a neurologist). They are both extremely satisfied with the condition of my hands and legs. After all, the fact that I cannot play the piano and that I can walk up steps only with the greatest of difficulty has no importance. One need not play the piano, and one can avoid going up steps and stairs. One can just sit at home, there is no need to traipse about slippery pavements and steps. Quite right: yesterday I went for a walk, fell over and banged my knee. Had I stayed at home this wouldn't have happened. And as for everything else, things are going excellently. As before, I can't smoke or drink. There have been temptations. But my foolish terror is stronger than any such temptations' [Wilson, 1994].

In her comprehensive biography 'Shostakovich: A Life', Laurel Fay [2000] notes,

'After eight years of consultations and treatments that had failed to produce a definitive diagnosis, let alone a cure, his cynicism was understandable. What was more remarkable, for all his afflictions and the steady physical deterioration, was the tenacity with which Shostakovich held on to the hope for improvement. Regularly he submitted to the tedium of lengthy hospital stays, medical consultations, myriad treatments and therapies. He consulted with specialists on his foreign trips. He tried exotic herbal preparations and alternative remedies; he thanked Shaginyan in January 1967, for instance, for her gift of a Japanese magnetic bracelet, saying he would wear it and try to believe in its miracle-working properties.'

Photographs from the mid-1960s tend to show Shostakovich using his left hand in conversation, during speeches, and while playing the piano. It is difficult to find photographs from this time in which he is using his right hand. Grigori Kozinstev, a director, met with Shostakovich in 1970 to discuss a film score. 'He limps, and can no longer play his music. He has been ill for a long time. His hand has shrivelled up, his bones are brittle ...'. [Wilson, 1994].

Shostakovich traveled to the USA in 1973 to accept an honorary doctorate from Northwestern University. During the trip, the composer received a two-day medical evaluation at the National Institute of Health in Bethesda, apparently confirming the conclusion that he suffered from a progressive incurable paralytic disorder (along with heart disease) [Fay, 2000].

Shostakovich provides details of his ailments in what turned out to be one of his final written intimations:

'There were no particularly happy moments in my life, no great joys. It was drab and dull and it makes me sad to think about it. Man feels joy when he's healthy and happy. I was often ill. I'm ill now, and my illness deprives me of the opportunity to take pleasure in ordinary things. It's hard for me to walk. I'm teaching myself to write with my left hand in case my right one gives out completely. I am utterly in the hands of the doctors, and I take all the medicine they prescribe, even if it sickens me. Now all they talk about is courage … when I'm in Moscow, I feel worst of all. I keep thinking that I'll fall and break a leg. I'm afraid to go out. I'm terrified of being seen, I feel so fragile, breakable…' [Jackson, 1997].

Solomon Volkov, a long-time acquaintance of Shostakovich, wrote 'Testimony', in which he records what he claims to be the memoirs of his friend. He paints a vivid portrait of Dmitri Dmitriyevich Shostakovich as nervous and fearful regarding his own mortality [Volkov, 1979]. His music of this final period expressed fear before death, a numbness, a search for a final sanctuary in the memory of future men; explosions of impotent and heartbreaking anger.

In the Kremlin hospital Shostakovich wrote his final letter:

'Dear Krzysztof: Thank you for remembering me, thank you for the letter. I am again in hospital, due to lung and heart problems. I manage to write with my right hand only with the greatest difficulty. Please excuse my scribbles. Best wishes to Zosia, a warm handshake. D. Shostakovich. P.S. Although it was very difficult for me I wrote a sonata for viola and piano' Wilson [1994].

Therefore, it appears that up until the end he could still use his right hand to some degree, at least enough to write notes and compose music. Also, the final letter illustrates that his intellectual function was preserved up until the end, which would be typical for most neuromuscular diseases.

Regarding Shostakovich's final days, Wilson [1994] writes:

'He stayed in hospital throughout July and came home on 1 August, very weakened. On 3 August, while eating a peach, he choked, and as a result of a prolonged attack of coughing which lasted several minutes, the malfunction of the heart got worse again. He was taken to hospital for a few days. Nothing however indicated that the end was near. On 9 August at 6:50 he unexpectedly started to suffocate ... The agony lasted for 40 minutes, and for the last 15 the composer was unconscious.'

It is possible that he choked on the peach simply as a coincidence leading to his decompensation. On the other hand, speech and swallowing weakness are common in ALS, and it could well be that he had impairment of swallowing with a tendency to choke (dysphagia) as a result of motor neuron disease. In addition, given the tendency for ALS patients to have diaphragmatic weakness, it could be that coincidental choking with subsequent aspiration pneumonia could lead to more severe decompensation.

Discussion

Such is the information available to us regarding Shostakovich's illness. While none of the major biographies of Shostakovich clearly state that he suffered from or was diagnosed with ALS, such a conclusion has made its way into the MDA and neuromuscular literature, as his name has been added to the substantial list of famous people who have had ALS [Pascuzzi, 1999].

A documented formal neurological examination would of course be required in order to reach a firm conclusion regarding the diagnosis of ALS [Pascuzzi, 2002]. His clinical course exceeded 15 years, while the majority of ALS patients have a more rapid progression with survival from onset of symptoms of 2–5 years. Yet, about 20% of ALS patients have a clinical course longer than 5 years and 10% have survival beyond 10 years. On the other hand the presence of a slow clinical course would raise the question of spinomuscular atrophy, and thus the significance of knowing results of a formal neurological examination. Typical ALS patients have upper motor neuron signs of spasticity and hyper-reflexia while spinomuscular atrophy is a pure lower motor neuron disease resulting in indolent atrophy and weakness. Another slow form of motor neuron disease is X-linked bulbo-spinomuscular atrophy or Kennedy's disease, a condition characterized by pure lower motor neuron disease, a slow course of progression, symmetrical limb weakness, atrophy and fasciculations of the face and tongue muscles, and gynecomastia as well as a family history consistent with an X-linked pattern of inheritance (males affected with the gene coming from the mother). The lack of a family history, the asymmetrical presentation would make this diagnosis unlikely. Could Shostakovich have suffered from multifocal motor neuropathy? Multifocal motor neuropathy is an inflammatory autoimmune disorder of particular interest in the differential diagnosis of Shostakovich, in that the clinical presentation can mimic slow motor neuron disease, can certainly evolve insidiously over 15–20 years and produce asymmetrical disabling limb weakness. The condition was not well recognized until the 1980s and thus would not have been considered by Shostakovich's physicians. Of all the diagnostic possibilities, multifocal motor neuropathy represents the most treatable (typically improving in response to intravenous γ-globulin). If his neurological examination confirmed the presence of upper motor neuron signs or the presence of bulbar deficits then multifocal motor neuropathy would be eliminated from the differential diagnosis. There is no evidence that he had paralytic polio and progressive symptoms from post-polio syndrome. Cervical myelopathy due to spondylosis, as well as syringomyelia are in the differential diagnosis. Inclusion body myositis can run a slow course, be asymmetric, and cause dysphagia [Pascuzzi, 2002]. Neurological examination would clarify some of these possibilities, and it would be interesting to see the results of myelography, nerve conduction studies and electromyography, assuming they were performed on the composer.

Shostakovich was a heavy smoker and suffered from coronary artery disease. He had heart attacks in the 1960s and 1970s. Additionally it is written that in his later years he suffered from lung cancer.

In spite of a slowly progressive paralytic disorder, lasting over 15 years, Shostakovich continued to compose music up until the time of his death. His remarkable cultural contributions, in the setting of a progressive disabling neurological condition, serve as an inspiration for other patients who are beset with chronic paralytic illness, including those with ALS.

Throughout his 68 years, Shostakovich achieved great triumph and suffered bitter disappointment. As a young man, his genius went largely unrecognized. It is unfortunate that, by the time he achieved international acclaim, he was so troubled with medical problems that he seems to have been unable to enjoy it. However, the legendary composer worked until his last days and his music remains a testament to a life of hardship and passion.

Shostakovich and ALS

Selected Quotations about Shostakovich – New York Times, April 12, 2002

Bernard Holland, Music Critic: 'With Shostakovich the division is between public and private. Any knowledge of Shostakovich on CD starts with the string quartets; 15 items that record a kind of secret diary stretched over a mature life. They can be horrifyingly sad and wickedly funny, but they speak in a language distinct to the composer. There is no other music like it.'

Paul Griffith: 'Many Shostakovichian paradoxes are knotted up within the Fifth Symphony, always explained as a piece the composer was forced to write. It is always admired as a work of tremendous personal authority. Ostensibly direct in expression with strong links to Russian music of the 19th century, it is fathomless in its ironies.'

Allan Kozinn: 'Shostakovich's concertos can be as melancholy as the symphonies and quartets, but by their nature they are also more lyrical. Now and then they are even bright and playful: listen to the second and last movements of the First Violin Concerto or the finale of the First Piano Concerto.'

Anthony Tommasini: 'After all the distress, sadness, and frenzy of Shostakovich's Fifth Symphony the final movement ends famously in an outburst of cosmic affirmation. Many listeners have found the affirmation forced.... This 1937 symphony was written in response to the denunciation of Shostakovich by Stalinist cultural committees the previous year, and the rejoicing is indeed forced. Shostakovich said: "It is as if someone were beating you with a stick and saying 'your business is rejoicing, your business is rejoicing'."

'The 15 string quartets … though mostly adhering to neoclassical structures, each quartet is such an affecting personal confession that you almost feel uncomfortable listening. It is like reading someone's private journals.'

Amyotrophic Lateral Sclerosis and Famous People

ALS has a prevalence of 1 in 10,000 people. Considering that the typical life expectancy for patients with ALS is 2–5 years, the lifetime chance for any person to develop ALS is approximately 1 in 700. It should therefore be logical that over history ALS has affected many famous individuals in all walks of life. If one looks at the number of well-known people in history who have had ALS, it helps confirm the notion that the disease is much more common than most people (including most physicians) appreciate. In addition to Shostakovich, jazz composer and musician Charles Mingus had ALS, as did the father of American folk music Huddy Ledbetter (Leadbelly). Many famous American athletes besides Lou Gehrig have been diagnosed with ALS: the great baseball pitcher James 'Catfish' Hunter; Bob Waters, Matt Hazeltine and Gary Lewis, 3 professional football players of the San Francisco 49'ers from the early 1960s, and the great heavyweight boxer from Cincinnati, Ezzard Charles (also known as the Cincinnati Cobra). Entertainers from the likes of David Niven and Dennis

Day had ALS. Dr. Stephen Hawking, the eminent physicist from England, has been assumed to have motor neuron disease and perhaps ALS. He became ill initially while in college, over 40 years ago. He is now in his mid-60s. The slow course would suggest a typically slower form of motor neuron disease such as spinomuscular atrophy. Another ALS patient is the physician Eliot Porter who received his MD degree from Harvard in 1929 and during World War II helped develop radar at MIT. Dr. Porter subsequently turned to a career of natural photography for which he is best known. Then, there is Henry Wallace who served as Secretary of Agriculture and also Vice-President of the United States under Franklin Roosevelt. Had Roosevelt not chosen to replace him with Harry Truman on the ticket for the 1944 election, Henry Wallace would have been President (since Roosevelt died 6 months after beginning his last term in office). Henry Wallace also had ALS. Mao Tse-Tung ('once all struggle is grasped, miracles are possible') is said to have had ALS as well. Therefore, as one looks around there is a remarkable list of individuals throughout history who have had ALS, which emphasizes the point that the disease is not as rare as most people think.

Selection of Quotations by Shostakovich

'A creative artist works on his next composition because he is not satisfied with his previous one' 1959.

'I always try to make myself as widely understood as possible; and if I don't succeed, I consider it my own fault.'

'Art destroys silence.'

'When a man is in despair, it means that he still believes in something.'

'I write music, it's performed. After all, my music says it all. It doesn't need historical and hysterical commentaries. In the long run, any words about music are less important than the music.'

'What you have in your head, put it down on paper. The head is a fragile vessel.'

'Every piece of music is a form of personal expression for its creator … If a work doesn't express the composer's own personal point of view, his own ideas, then it doesn't, in my opinion, even deserve to be born' 1973.

References

Fay LE: Shostakovich: A Life. New York, Oxford University Press, 2000.
Jackson S: Dmitri Shostakovich. An Essential Guide to His Life and Works. Classic FM Lifelines. London, Pavilion Books, 1997.
Pascuzzi RM: Shostakovich and amyotrophic lateral sclerosis. Semin Neurol 1999;19(suppl 1):63–66.
Pascuzzi RM: ALS, motor neuron disease, and related disorders: a personal approach to diagnosis and management. Semin Neurol 2002;22:75–87.

Varzar IV: The Last Summer Together. Translated for DSCH by Joan Pemberton Smith. DSCH Journal No. 2, Winter 1994.

Volkov S: Testimony. The Memoirs of Dmitri Shostakovich. Translated from the Russian by Antonina W. Bouis. New York, Harper & Row, 1979.

White RH: Shostakovich versus the Central Committee: the power of music. Clin Med 2008;8:405–409.

Wilson E: Shostakovich. A Life Remembered. Princeton, Princeton University Press, 1994.

Robert M. Pascuzzi, MD, Professor and Chair of Neurology
Indiana University School of Medicine, Indiana Clinic, Clarian Health
Department of Neurology
Emerson Hall 125, 545 Barnhill Drive, Indianapolis, IN 46202 (USA)
Tel. +1 317 274 4455, E-Mail rpascuzz@iupui.edu

Bogousslavsky J, Hennerici MG, Bäzner H, Bassetti C (eds): Neurological Disorders in Famous Artists – Part 3. Front Neurol Neurosci. Basel, Karger, 2010, vol 27, pp 101–118

....

Suffering for Her Art: The Chronic Pain Syndrome of Pianist Clara Wieck-Schumann

Eckart Altenmüller[a], *Reinhard Kopiez*[b]

[a]Institut für Musikphysiologie und Musiker-Medizin, und [b]Institut für musikpädagogische Forschung, Hochschule für Musik und Theater Hannover, Hannover, Germany

Abstract

Clara Schumann was an outstanding pianist, systematically trained as a child prodigy by her father Friedrich Wieck. Married to the composer Robert Schumann she gave birth to 8 children, however, was able to continue performing regularly in public. After the mental breakdown of her husband, she had to increase her public performance activities due to the need to earn a living for her large family. In this time, the first pains in the right arm occurred, which at the beginning were of shorter duration, however increasingly required prolonged periods of rest. Later, when attempting to work on the highly demanding piano works of Johannes Brahms, especially on his first piano concerto, she developed chronic pain, which forced her to interrupt any concert activities for more than 1 year. Obviously, Brahms' modern treatment of the piano in an almost orchestral way imposed technical difficulties which Clara Schumann was not properly prepared to deal with. Finally, she underwent a multimodal pain therapy in the private sanatorium of Dr. Esmarch, which consisted of an integrated interdisciplinary approach comprising pain medication, psychotherapy, physiotherapy and modification of playing habits. She fully recovered and successfully continued her career as an internationally renowned concert pianist. The case report impressively demonstrates the stressors an outstanding female elite musician had to cope with in the 19th century. Furthermore, it is a convincing example of how the intuition and mere experience of a sensitive and understanding doctor lead to the right conclusions and to a modern multimodal pain therapy in chronic overuse injury. Furthermore the case report demonstrates the important role of prevention, including physical exercises, self-awareness, and reasonable practice schedules.

Copyright © 2010 S. Karger AG, Basel

This chapter is a modified and shortened translation of an article which appeared in German in the book: 'Krankheiten grosser Musiker und Musikerinnen: Reflexionen am Schnittpunkt von Musikwissenschaft und Medizin', Altenmüller E, Rode-Breymann S (eds), Hildesheim, Olms, 2009.

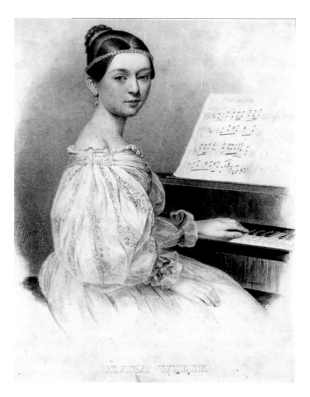

Fig. 1. Clara Wieck. Lithograph, Hannover 1835, by Julius Glière. Visible on the music rest is the beginning of the third movement of Clara's Piano Concerto in A. Reprinted with kind permission, Robert-Schumann-Haus, Zwickau.

'Imagine, I had only just arrived when I felt such pains in my left arm that I had a terrible night and the next morning I had to cancel the concert and journey back, then I had to cancel another concert and various other things here.'

Clara Schumann in a letter to Joseph Joachim dated November 27, 1857 [Litzmann, 1923, vol I, p 26).

In Germany, Clara Schumann (fig. 1) is remembered with affection as the attractive young woman with the double-parted curls who gazes romantically out from the old 100-D-Mark notes. To many Germans, she was the loyal wife of composer Robert Schumann, who died at the age of 46. But what is less well known is that she was a composer in her own right and also an outstanding pianist, who was one of the first women ever to play concert tours all over Europe. If she were alive today, she would be an international star like Martha Argerich. But Clara Wieck-Schumann's wonderful performances came at a price: her schedule was constantly interrupted because of periods of ill health caused by pain in her arms.

This chapter looks at the pain caused by playing the piano. What were the circumstances leading up to this pain? Did Clara Schumann suffer from a chronic rheumatic disease, as her doctors suspected? Or were the pains largely psychosomatic, brought on by the many stress factors in her life: the excessive demands placed on her by caring for a large family; the long, uncomfortable journeys, and the constant financial worries? Did the pains arise specifically because she was a pianist – were they signs of overload caused by too much practicing and playing? Were contemporary composers such as Johannes Brahms making new demands in terms of technique which were physically too much for Clara Schumann?

We will be making a detailed analysis of these questions with the help of musical biography, expert research and modern-day doctors who specialize in musicians' injuries. In this way we would like to demonstrate how Clara's medical problems typically reflect the darker side of virtuosity, specialization and the modern concert scene. Pain disorders caused by playing an instrument have always been a common problem, and continue to be so to the present day. The most comprehensive study of this topic was carried out in the USA by Fishbein and Middlestadt [1988]. They ran a survey of 4,025 professionally performing musicians from 48 American orchestras in which they asked specific questions about pain disorders. A total of 2,212 musicians responded to the survey. Of these, 76% stated they had 'serious problems' which affected their playing. 49% of those with 'serious problems' suffered musculoskeletal pain, its actual location depending on the instrument played and the particular strain involved. Violinists typically had problems with shoulders and arms, while cellists and wind players were generally affected in the neck and back [for a review see, Altenmüller and Jabusch, 2008].

Another study of young pianists showed a lifetime prevalence of 25% for pain syndromes which required at least 2 days away from the instrument [Shields and Dockrell, 2000]. The sheer volume of ailments is astonishing, but it seems that incidental pain when playing is an everyday occurrence for most musicians. So it is not surprising that Joseph Joachim, recipient of the above-quoted letter dated December 1, 1857, should reply by trying to comfort her with the following anecdote:

'My poor dear friend, you have had so much to bear – having to exist alone without music. How terrible! The same thing happened to me 4 years ago, just after I had taken up my new position of concertmaster. During our first rehearsal of Mendelssohn's symphony, which should have been my first performance, I strained myself because of my excessive fervor and for the next two weeks I could lift neither bow nor pen – what a debut for me when I had no acquaintances and no support from my fellow-players!' [Litzmann, 1923, vol I, p 28].

Clara Wieck's Musical Training

It is worth taking a closer look at the training which Clara received from her father, Friedrich Wieck. What methods did he use to enable her to gain international recognition and to develop Clara's resilience, technical perfection, creativity and spontaneity? In his teaching did he in fact use knowledge of 'music physiology'?

Friedrich Wieck was born in 1785 in Pretzsch an der Elbe, about 45 km from Leipzig. His parents were merchants, but business was not good and they lived in humble circumstances. Friedrich was passionate about music from an early age, and was particularly interested in piano technique. However, he followed his parents' wishes and first studied theology, though he was never appointed to a parish. Instead he took a position as tutor for Baron Seckendorff in Querfurth, and he became friends with the musician Adolph Bargiel, who was later to marry Wieck's first wife.

One of Friedrich Wieck's striking characteristics was his interest in pedagogical matters. He had read the educational treatises of Johann Heinrich Pestalozzi and Jean-Jacques Rousseau and later used their main pedagogic principles in his piano teaching. In 1815 he opened a music shop and educational establishment in Leipzig (today it would be called a 'private music school') where he taught piano and music theory and his wife Marianne also taught piano, as well as giving singing lessons. Here he was able to develop his pedagogical interests and begin to use them to aid the progress of his daughter Clara [for a review see, de Vries, 1996].

Clara Wieck was born on September 13, 1819. By the age of four she was playing melodies and short pieces on the piano by ear. When she turned five, her father started her on his 'complete' musical training, which did not simply concentrate on finger dexterity but encompassed the development of musical expression, singing, and the avoidance of excessive tension. Wieck taught her how to play with great expression while keeping her wrists and elbows relaxed and using the greatest possible economy of movement [Köckritz, 2007; Klassen, 2009]. Her flawless legato and 'song-like' melodic lines attracted the admiration of the famous violinist and composer Louis Spohr, who was amazed by the consummate smoothness of 12-year-old Clara's playing and attested that she 'made the instruments sound more beautiful' [Walch-Schumann, 1968].

Another important principle of the training was the avoidance of physical and mental exhaustion. So as a child, Clara was allowed to practice piano for no more than 3 h/day, and she had to spend at least the same amount of time exercising outside in the fresh air. Friedrich Wieck's method also included physical exercises to improve playing technique, such as specific finger-stretching exercises to increase the span of Clara's hand. Indeed, later on Clara was able to play tenths with a loose wrist and also included wide-spanning chords in her own compositions.

Once Clara was 7 years old, the 'complete' training method was supplemented with a thorough schooling in music theory. She received lessons in music theory, counterpoint and composition, and regularly attended concerts by the Gewandhaus orchestra, as well as visits to the Leipzig opera house and theater. And in order to develop her own teaching skills, when she was 11 years old she was assigned the task of teaching her younger brother Alwin to play the piano [Steegmann, 2001].

Up to the age of 12, Clara's repertoire consisted mainly of 'virtuoso, popular, brilliant pieces which were in currency at the time' as Monica Steegmann [2001] describes in her biography of Clara Schumann. It was dominated by the works of Hummel, Moscheles, Czerny, Herz, Kalkbrenner und Field. But from 1833 onwards a canonized repertoire, as described by Kopiez et al. [2009] was already becoming established. It was now dominated by Chopin, Mendelssohn, Robert Schumann and Beethoven, but their works did not really conform to popular taste at the time and their compositions were considered avant-garde. We are fortunate enough to have detailed knowledge of Clara Schumann's repertoires. Litzmann [1923] gives a chronological listing of Clara's study pieces and repertoire from page 615 onwards in volume 3 of his above-mentioned biography. We also have at our disposal a complete set of her 1,312 concert programs, which have recently been critically analyzed using statistical methods [Kopiez et al., 2009].

In conclusion, Clara Schumann's training as a pianist was developed in accordance with remarkably modern considerations relating to music physiology. Limiting daily practice to 3 h, avoiding monotonous, purely mechanical finger exercises, bringing diverse aspects of musical theory into the training, paying attention to health issues by promoting stretching exercises and regular walks in the fresh air – what we would today call 'mild endurance training' – all these are pedagogic principles which can help to develop great resilience and an accelerated rate of learning [Altenmüller and McPherson, 2007]. In this way, Friedrich Wieck was a step ahead of his contemporaries, who overemphasized the value of long hours of practice. Even as children, the pianists Clementi and Czerny were spending 8 h/day in 'solitary confinement' at their pianos, while Kalkbrenner was practicing 12 h and Henselt as much as 16 h/day. However, leading performers and teachers reacted to such feats of endurance with a note of irony. In the foreword to his 1811 piano tutor, Hummel writes: 'I can assure you that regular, attentive practice of at most three hours per day is sufficient; longer practice dulls the spirit and leads to playing which is machine-like rather than soulful' [quoted according to Gellrich, 1992].

Stresses and Strains of Piano Playing

Systematically building an international career as a pianist required – and still requires today – great physical and mental resilience. From the age of 11 Clara went on regular concert tours which placed her under enormous stress. Friedrich Wieck's letters are full of complaints about uncomfortable carriages, poor accommodation, defective instruments and local complications [Walch-Schumann, 1968]. It is clear that there was no respite for Clara: in a letter from her father to his wife dated February 20, 1837, he describes the triumph of her concert in Berlin and then adds: 'Clara is suffering with her eyes because of the brightness of the lights, and almost all her nails have split – but her fingers do not hurt. …' Clara was obviously extremely resilient in terms of her piano playing because of the solid training she had received from her father, her clever choice of repertoire and her optimal practice technique. For example, she withstood the heavy demands of her first stay in Vienna from November 1837 to April 1838, where she played up to three concerts or private recitals every day, without adverse effects on her health. And this was despite the enormous emotional pressure caused by the intensive exchange of letters she was having with her suitor Robert Schumann, which she was keeping secret from her father. The diaries and letters of Clara and her father up to 1857 show no clear evidence of overuse injuries caused by playing. Nevertheless, her physical wellbeing was always a concern. On September 16, 1836 Clara took a fall while on her way to a concert in Naumburg. In Litzmann [1923, vol I, p 106] we find the following account:

'It could have been a day of great misfortune for Clara. She took a tumble on her way to the concert … as a result her left hand swelled up hugely and caused her severe pain for several days.'

Wieck talks unequivocally about this event:

'We were on our tour of the cities, and in Naumburg the sword of Damocles hung over her precious head.'

There is also no evidence in later years of any ailments, even short-term ones that restricted her ability to perform, particularly as Clara's concert appearances became much less frequent after her marriage to Robert Schumann in 1840. Before her marriage, from 1828 to 1840, Clara averaged 17 concerts per season, while after her marriage, in the years 1840 to 1854, she averaged 10 concerts per season, the number of concerts varying between 22 (season 1844/45) and 4 (season 1845/46), due to her confinements [Kopiez et al., 2009, fig. 3]. It should be noted that Clara Schumann bore eight children and had two miscarriages between 1841 and 1854.

It is not hard to imagine the tremendous strain that Clara must have been under at that time. The large Schumann household found themselves under constant financial pressure and they needed her successful concert performances in order to survive. But the demands of running the household, supporting her husband and organizing her own concerts – without the help of her father – meant that Clara had no time to regularly work on her repertoire. This came to the fore during her second trip to Vienna at the end of 1846. Clara travelled there with her husband and their two eldest daughters, 5-year-old Marie and 3-year old Elise, and she organized her own concerts there. Before the third concert she wrote: 'I feel like a hunted animal. I only had one hour to prepare for the concert. I fear tomorrow's concert will be unremarkable' [Wendler 1996].

Clara's responsibilities increased still more after her husband was admitted to hospital in Endenich on March 4, 1854. Now Clara not only had to earn a living to support herself and her 7 surviving children (her son Emil, born 1846, died 1 year later), but she also had to cover the high costs of Robert Schumann's treatment at the clinic. So in October 1854 she undertook her first long concert tour since her marriage, playing 22 concerts in the months before Christmas.

It was during this more intensive period of public performances that she first began to feel more persistent pain, which was clearly brought on by playing the piano.

Onset of Overuse Problems due to Playing the Piano

The circumstances surrounding the onset of the more persistent pains which Clara Schumann felt in her left arm are typical of overuse injuries. In her letter to Joseph Joachim of November 27, 1857, quoted earlier, Clara herself alluded to them:

'On the morning of the day when my problems began, I had another very enjoyable rehearsal with the orchestra. I was supposed to play Robert's concerto but I really overreached myself. I have never felt such a sense of enthusiasm emanating from the orchestra as after this concerto; I felt it penetrate to my core and I also became so inspired that I totally forgot myself and everything which lay ahead of me.'

Clara was obviously in that positive emotional state which can be termed as 'flow' [Czikszentmihalyi, 1990] and in this inspired condition she was not aware of the physical signals which were warning her of overload. It is well known that the release of endorphins linked to a flow experience can cause pain to be suppressed [Suaudeau and Costentin, 2000]. On top of that, rehearsals are always particularly physically demanding for orchestral soloists. The requirement to be heard against the sound of the orchestra can easily lead to a forced style of playing, and, unlike in solo practice, the time spent playing is controlled by the conductor, meaning that necessary breaks are often not taken.

Medical studies show another typical factor which often leads to the onset of pain, namely general physical debility due to an infection. In the above-mentioned letter we read:

'A medical examination has shown that the problem was a rheumatic inflammation, caused partly by excessive strain and partly by a head cold' [Litzmann 1923, vol III, p 27].

Treatment of the pain largely followed the same principles as modern-day treatment. Clara was given a strong analgesic in the form of opium, she was ordered to rest from playing and her arm was immobilized in a sling. The symptoms quickly improved but flared up again 10 days later, understandably causing her considerable concern. On December 6 she wrote in her diary: 'Sleepless night, very afraid that I will have to return home because of the pains in my arm which are getting worse and worse' [Litzmann 1923, vol III, p 29]. Nowadays we know that worrying about pain actually increases the likelihood of it becoming chronic. A pain is described as chronic if it lasts for longer than 3 months. It is not quite clear how long Clara suffered from pain in her left arm, but it seems it was still plaguing her in early 1858, for Johannes Brahms writes to her in a letter dated February 24: 'I cannot wait until I hear from you. I have to learn patience due to your injured arm and probably also the agitation about the concerts' [Litzmann, 1927, vol I, p 216]. However it seems unlikely that the pain was chronic at this time, as at the end of December 1857 Clara was performing some very difficult works, including on December 19 Robert Schumann's 'Symphonic Studies' in Zurich and on December 25 his piano concerto in Munich. From January 27, 1858, Clara was once again on tour in Switzerland and there is no mention of any health problems in her letters or diaries.

The Perils of a Demanding Repertoire

In the years that followed, Clara extended her repertoire. In the autumn of 1861 she rehearsed Brahms' Händel Variations Op. 24, writing about them to her daughter Marie: 'they are terribly difficult, but I have just about learned them' [Litzmann 1923, vol III, p 111]. She recounts in her diary her first public performance of them on December 7 of that year: 'I was scared to death while playing them, but I was successful and received loud applause' [Litzmann 1923, vol III, p 112].

On December 3, 1861, she performed for the first time Brahms' Piano Concerto No. 1 in D minor, conducted by Brahms himself, in Hamburg. Clara noted in her diary:

'… I was probably the happiest person in the whole hall, because although it was physically demanding and I was very nervous, everything was outweighed by my enjoyment of

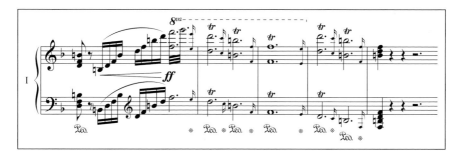

Fig. 2. Johannes Brahms, Piano Concerto in D minor Op. 15. Even today, the formidable octave trills in the first movement present a challenge for pianists.

the piece and the fact that he was conducting it himself. I was not even irritated by the stupid audience who understood nothing and felt nothing ...' [Litzmann 1923, vol III, p 112].

In February 1858 Brahms wrote to Clara shortly after completing this work: 'I have been practicing the first movement furiously. I do not think you will be able to sustain it. But I would love just once to hear you play the Adagio and Rondo in public' [Litzmann 1927, vol I, p 219].

Brahms was obviously aware of the difficulties presented by this piano composition. In particular, the formidable fortissimo octave trills in the first movement required a new wide-spanning 'shaking movement' of the forearms, a technique which Clara had never tried before (fig. 2). But he underestimated the enthusiasm and sheer willpower of his loyal friend and supporter – she was not to be denied the opportunity to perform it in Brahms' hometown.

Although Clara retained a life-long love of Brahms' compositions, she avoided performing them in public in the years that followed. She felt that these piano works were too much for her physically. This is why she performed Brahms' works quite rarely compared to other composers in her repertoire: Brahms lay in 7th place with 2.3%, behind Schumann (28.4%), Mendelssohn (12.0%), Beethoven (11.5%), Chopin (10.8%), Schubert (6.9%) und Bach (3.1%) [Kopiez et al., 2009, fig 1c]. She only twice performed his Piano Concerto No. 1, whereas she gave public performances of her husband's concerto (Op. 54) 110 times, Beethoven's Piano Concerto No. 4 (Op. 58) 59 times, and Mendelssohn's Piano Concerto No. 1 (Op. 25) 56 times.

Clara explicitly refers to these excessive physical demands in a letter to Brahms written in London on April 8, 1871, during her English concert tour:

'... then my fatigued muscles played a trick on me – I did not dare to attempt such an arduous piece, as I had to play three times a week, which required of me a great deal of energy. The problem lay with your Händel Variations, which I absolutely wanted to include in my recital but which in the end I had to admit were too hard for me. I am unspeakably sad that these Variations which I love so much are simply beyond me' [Litzmann, 1927, vol I, p 639].

From early 1872 onwards, we see more and more evidence of her ailments. The excessive demands of her annual English tour caused the symptoms to reappear. While in London she wrote a letter to Brahms dated February 21, 1872, in which she says:

'I have good news for you in that I am being afforded an enthusiastic reception, people say I have never played so well, etc.; but I am suffering terribly with rheumatism in my arm and finger muscles, so that I am quite afraid to look ahead from one engagement to the next. Although I am practicing everything pianissimo, I am still absolutely exhausted after an hour – of course the rheumatism is afflicting the parts which are under the most strain' [Litzmann, 1927, vol II, p 6].

So first of all Clara reduced the volume when practicing, but practice sessions of 1 h (probably without a break) would still be considered too long when measured by today's medical criteria relating to musicians. Interestingly, the 'enthusiastic reception' mentioned in this passage was in respect to a work by Brahms, namely his arrangement of the Gavotte after Gluck [Litzmann, 1923, vol III, p 272]. It is not clear whether the uncomfortable 'Brahmsian' movement in the arrangement was too much for Clara, but a few days later she wrote in another letter:

'I have just requested your Hungarian duets from Simrock – I wonder whether I will be able to master any of them?' [Litzmann, 1927, vol I, p 8].

Clearly, these works with wide-spanning chords which necessitated an excellent leap and octave technique were also a challenge for Clara. But she was also worried about other playing techniques, as evidenced in a letter to her friend in Hamburg, the pianist Theodor Avé-Lallement, concerning the students at the Stuttgart Conservatory:

'… firstly, as a matter of principle, I do not accept any students from the Stuttgart Conservatory, because I do not approve of their technique and no matter how hard I try I cannot eradicate it from their playing. … their fingers are like storks' legs walking up and down the piano and the worst thing is that they are compromising their health by practicing in this way: most of them become nervous and develop weak fingers or weak chests. This outcome is inevitable; I only have to play in this way for a few moments before I get terrible pains in my arm muscles' [Litzmann, 1923, vol III, p 276].

This once again shows how Clara looked at things very much from a physiological standpoint – in this respect she was very much her father's loyal student. By 'storks' legs' she probably means exaggerated widely stretched finger movements which disregard the weight of the arm and the flexibility of the wrist.

After the summer break, during the 1872/1873 season there is no mention of any pain. But it may be that Clara was preoccupied by other sad events. Her daughter Julie was in her third pregnancy and seriously ill with tuberculosis. In August she came to the Schumann family house in Baden-Baden with her husband and eldest son, and on November 10 she died of her illness. As was the case later on when her son Felix died, Clara was away on a concert tour when she received the sad news, but she continued with her engagements. Once again we see evidence not only of her enormous self-discipline and will-power, but also her professional desire not to disappoint her public or let down her fellow musicians.

In winter 1872 she was still suffering from physical problems when playing the piano, as is shown in a letter she wrote to Brahms from London dated March 6, 1873:

'Now I would so love to be able to play the Händel Variations, but I can hardly practice at all. I will just be happy if I can get through the concerts, for the pains in my hands and arms are becoming so bad that I am often seriously worried' [Litzmann, 1927, vol I, p 15].

We once again see evidence of the difficulties presented by Brahms' works. Her doctor advised her to avoid writing, which suggests that her right hand was most badly affected. On April 12 she wrote in a letter from London:

'… by being extremely cautious I was able to fulfill all my engagements: I only ever practiced at half volume and did not do any writing. I was very happy that I managed to get through them, but during the final engagement last Monday I could only move my fingers. I could no longer lift my arms and I needed poultices for the rest of the week. I have now started with homeopathic treatment, which is supposed to be very effective for this kind of pain' [Litzmann, 1927, vol I, p 16].

Today we would say that it was high time she took a break from playing, but she did not cancel her concerts, indeed she planned a final matinee performance on April 26. But in order to give her hand a little respite, Clara began to dictate some of her correspondence. On November 24, 1873 she dictated a letter to Brahms:

'… my hand and arm joints are really painful so I am dictating almost everything' [Litzmann, 1927, vol I, p 16].

In view of her poor health it was quite amazing that Clara risked performing for the second (and last) time Brahms' Piano Concerto No. 1 in D minor at the Leipzig Gewandhaus on December 3. It was a pyrrhic victory, for in a letter to Brahms dated December 12, 1873, she wrote

'Your concerto has given me so many pleasant, even happy, hours. It is so beautiful and I performed it successfully in Leipzig … I would need to play it every year, another 3–4 times, so that the audiences could also become familiar with it. But who knows whether I will ever play it again, for the pains in my arm are now very bad – at the moment I cannot play at all, and indeed I should not be writing' [Litzmann, 1927, vol I, p 32].

Finally – A Consistent Treatment Regime

After her concerts in Leipzig, Clara finally decided to seek out a consistent treatment regime for her now chronic pain. For the first time in her long artistic career she took a break from playing and performing from mid-December 1873 to March 1875. She cancelled her tour of England and refused an invitation to play 100 concerts in America, and 'The piano has been closed for weeks – that is so hard!' [Litzmann 1927, vol I, p 41].

Her diagnosis was now reviewed, and according to the Berlin doctors it was not 'rheumatism', but 'overstimulation of the muscles'. From February 1874 her arm was treated using:

'A stroking and kneading treatment from a lady who has had considerable success with other patients. She thinks she will be able to help me recover, but I have to be patient because the pains are of a long-standing and persistent nature. … Of course at the beginning it was very painful' [Litzmann, 1927, vol I, p 41].

This treatment is probably very close to 'classic massage therapy', which today is still one of the standard methods used by physiotherapists to treat chronic muscular tension and pain. But unfortunately the treatment was not successful. In May, Clara went to Teplitz for 6 weeks of rehabilitation therapy. The pain in her arm meant she still had to dictate her letters and refrain from playing the piano. In particular this long period away from the piano seemed to gradually drive her to depression. Clara wrote in her diary on New Year's Eve 1874:

'A sad New Year's Eve – this year has been a difficult one for me and my travails are not yet over. I have not been able to practice my art, my consolation in difficult times. How hard it has been!' [Litzmann, 1923, vol III, p 316].

At the end of January 1875 Clara went to Kiel to be treated by the renowned surgeon Friedrich von Esmarch, who treated chronic pain syndrome in a very modern way even by today's standards. Clara wrote in her diary:

'I began the treatment on 27 (January), which consisted of massage, which was very painful at first but which improved after a few weeks, and douches. … Even on the first day I had to play piano for an hour, despite the pain – Esmarch insisted on this, whereas all the other doctors had strongly recommended rest – and the pains did not get worse as a result of it … Esmarch and his wife (the Princess of Schleswig-Holstein) are very kind people. Whenever he left (he visited me every morning) I felt happier than before he came. … The pains in my arm improved a little, though not significantly, it was painful to play, but I played nonetheless, I now had the courage to do it – it was also a kind of treatment for the mind … they tried to persuade me to play a concert, which at first really terrified me … but Esmarch quickly brought the matter to a head when he said he was going to write a prescription for me – "Play a concert", he needed to see how I coped with playing in public … On March 18 I gave my first concert for nearly 18 months. It went very well and everyone was very sympathetic. Among many beautiful flowers I received an anonymous bouquet from Berlin with the words:

Play without pain
Heartfelt wishes
A Berlin admirer' [Litzmann, 1923, vol III, p 318].

Esmarch was successful with his combination of physiotherapy, supportive psychotherapy and a cautious return to the piano. He can be considered to be the first of those modern-day doctors who specialize in musicians' injuries. He utilized a multi-dimensional, holistic pain therapy which is still in use today. The main elements of this therapy are:

(1) Release of muscle tension through physiotherapy and massage.
(2) Psychotherapeutic treatment of the accompanying anxiety and negative self-image which is often observed in these cases, along with the patient's loss of confidence in their own abilities.
(3) Promoting positive experiences at the instrument through resumed playing, systematic, structured training and through encouraging the patient to temporarily ignore the pain. In this way the negative associations which have been stored in the central nervous system relating to playing the instrument and the pain are gradually erased and the pain memory is 'overwritten'.

Admittedly, Clara was not now totally free of pain, but in the years that followed she understood how to avoid overstraining herself by paying attention to her choice of repertoire, planning her concerts carefully and making sure she took sufficient respites. It is interesting to see how this affected her playing of Johannes Brahms' works: in the 1872–1873 season, 2 years before her break from playing, she performed an unusually high number of works by Brahms, making up 9.3% of her repertoire. When her condition was at its worst during the season of 1873–1875 and even after her recovery in 1876–1877 she never again performed one of his works. After recovering from her chronic pain syndrome she obviously decided to avoid playing Brahms' potentially hazardous works.

Her health may also have improved because of the inner serenity she had achieved and the more secure financial situation she found herself in due to her appointment as teacher at the Hoch Conservatory in Frankfurt and the growing royalty income from her husband's works. Her friends also showed a tender concern for her health. A final example is the story of how Brahms came to arrange Johann Sebastian Bach's violin Chaconne in D minor for the piano left-hand:

'Dear Clara,
I think it is a long time since I have sent you anything [the arrangement of Bach's Chaconne for the left hand, ed.] as enjoyable as this – if your fingers can withstand the enjoyment! The Chaconne is one of the most wonderful, unfathomable pieces of music. ... Try it out, I have written it for you. But do not overstrain your hand! It requires a great deal of

sound and power, for the time being just play it mezza voce. But make sure the finger positions are manageable and comfortable …' [Litzmann, 1927, vol II, p 111].

Clara replied on July 6:

'Dearest Johannes,
That was certainly a wonderful surprise! It was really strange – on the day after my arrival I pulled a tendon in my right hand while I was opening a drawer, but the Chaconne has now become a real refuge for me. Only you could do such a thing … Admittedly, my fingers cannot quite sustain it, at the part with the repetition of the chords (notation of four repeated d-minor chords in octave distance consisting of quarter notes, [authors]). I always break down and my right hand too almost goes into cramp, but otherwise there are no insurmountable difficulties and I am taking great pleasure in it'. [Litzmann, 1927, vol II, p 112].

Diagnostic Classification

At first, Clara Schumann's condition is identified as 'rheumatism' by herself in her letters and diary entries and by the doctors who treated her. In the 19th century this term was often used to describe all forms of musculoskeletal pain, and does not mean that it was a rheumatic disorder in the modern sense of the word. The term 'rheumatism' was coined as early as 1683 by the Parisian doctor Guillaume de Baillou to describe what we now call rheumatoid arthritis. Over the following centuries, the meaning of the term expanded so that gout, prolapsed discs and other neuralgic pain was referred to as 'rheumatism' [for a review see, Gerabek et al., 2005].

It is always challenging to make a precise posthumous diagnosis, as the critical criteria for the diagnosis are normally not available. In Clara's day it was not possible to detect signs of inflammation through blood tests or to take X-rays of the fingers and arms. But rheumatoid arthritis seems unlikely, as there is no evidence of the symptoms included in the Criteria for Rheumatoid Arthritis as classified by the American College of Rheumatology: swelling or reddening of the joints, morning stiffness, pain occurring mainly in the mornings and at night, and rheumatic nodules [Hammer, 2006].

Diagnostically all the signs point to a chronic myofascial pain syndrome linked to overuse. This term describes pain which is caused by excessive strain on muscles, tendons, joints and soft connective tissues and which is characterized by tight muscles and dull, often shifting pains which get worse on exertion. No abnormalities show up in laboratory tests or X-rays. Characteristic symptoms include painful trigger points, particularly at tendon insertion points. The pains that Clara felt during her 'kneading treatments' suggest that she had these trigger points. The diagnosis of 'overstimulation of the muscles' which was made in Berlin in 1874 also fits in with this diagnosis.

Myofascial pain syndrome linked to overuse is by far the most common medical condition suffered by musicians and, more specifically, by pianists. The pain normally occurs in that part of the body which is put under strain due to repetitive movements over a long period. So pianists typically suffer from pain in the forearms, hands and finger joints, and occasionally also in the upper arms and shoulders. Clara Schumann also had problems in these areas. The pain is normally set off by overuse and at first is only felt while playing the instrument. There is evidence that this was Clara's experience. The pain is often not felt during everyday activities. It is triggered by extended periods of playing while preparing for important concerts and practicing unaccustomed techniques under time pressure. These were also clearly factors for Clara Schumann, if we think of the unfamiliar technique required to play the Brahms' piano concerto. Sometimes, after a certain age, pain can suddenly occur during particular playing actions which were never previously a problem. This pain can be attributed to diminished physical capacity and cumulative damage to the affected areas. Along with longer, more intensive playing sessions and practicing new exercises, non-musical activities such as writing can cause myofascial pain. Clara's medical history has abundant evidence of this too. Infections, mental strain and depression also increase susceptibility to chronic pain syndromes [for a review on this topic see, Brandfonbremer and Kjelland, 2002].

A Musical-Medical Assessment

How would Clara's ailments be treated today? Acute overuse injuries are very common and generally do not require any specific medical treatment. A few days rest, cold or heat treatment and careful stretching exercises are all that is needed for the majority of these injuries to clear up very quickly. If the pain lasts longer than 3 days, then non-steroidal anti-inflammatories should be taken under a doctor's supervision. Clara Schumann's pains lasted longer than 3 months, so we must assume they had become chronic. Our understanding of chronic pain has changed over the last decades. Nowadays it is believed that chronic pain is mainly due to maladaptive central nervous plasticity. Via increasing efficiency of synaptic transmission in the dorsal horn of the vertebral column and downregulation of pain-inhibiting circuits, persistent pain leads to increased afferent inflow to the thalamus and the more centrally located neural networks relevant for pain processing [for a review see, Fields and Basbaum, 1999]. Moreover, the anxiety caused by what is perceived as a serious pain event – which Clara clearly experienced – promotes a change in the somatosensory representation of the painful limb in the parietal cortex. According to Flor et al. [1997] and Tinazzi et al. [2000] as a correlate of chronic back or hand pain, the homuncular topography is distorted, enlarged and dedifferentiated. Obviously, this prominent change in neural representations correlates to pain memory. Typical for pains, related to such an associative network of pain-memory, symptoms mostly arise when playing and they occur in different locations and in different forms. A crucial part of therapy is to allay the patients' anxieties in order to break the vicious circle of feeling under threat and the pain becoming fixed in the pain memory. The sufferer should once again start to play their instrument, and it has been shown at first it is best to play for no more than 10 min at a time, several times a day. Clara's doctor Friedrich Esmarch used these basic treatment principles. In terms of medical history, this is a very fine example of how an effective therapy can be developed through intuition and empiricism, 100 years before the inception of experimental pain physiology and theories about how the central nervous system deals with pain.

Coda

Clara Wieck-Schumann's medical history is instructive in many ways. She received excellent training from her father and developed a technique which was both economical and physiologically sound. Unlike her husband Robert, in her youth she was not inclined towards compulsive overworking, a self-destructive lifestyle, nor to making excessive demands on herself [for a review of Robert Schumanns' compulsive working behavior see, Altenmüller, 2005]. She instead adopted a forward-looking, considered, very sound style of working. She was extremely resilient and even when under great pressure – such as during her second trip to Vienna – she was capable of performing at a high level. It is hardly an exaggeration to say that it is quite amazing how she stayed healthy for so long! This was thanks to her strong physical constitution and excellent training.

So what was the cause of her problems? We believe that the demands of Johannes Brahms' new style of playing were a prominent factor in causing the overstrain. This style, which as Robert Schumann said: 'transformed the piano into an orchestra of wailing and jubilant voices' [Schumann, 1962], was a new pianistic hurdle for Clara to overcome. She had grown up with the fluent technique of Hummel, Moscheles, Chopin and Mendelssohn, and was now confronted by pianistic problems to which she had no solution. At the same time she was facing a dilemma, for in her role as an influential artist she particularly wanted to promote this young composer. This was her motivation for performing his Piano Concerto No. 1 – with the consequences described. Social stresses, her tendency to anxiety, and the often adverse external circumstances surrounding her also contributed to the pain becoming chronic.

From a musical-medical point of view this is a unique case, because we are fortunate enough to have at our disposal source material which allows us to trace every small detail of a major historic artist's case history. The onset of pain, the various courses it took, the desperate efforts to fulfill all her concert commitments, the vain search for a 'fast' cure, and finally her patient rehabilitation under the aegis of an empathetic doctor are so clearly described and at the same time are so typical that every textbook of musical medicine should mention Clara Wieck-Schumann's case as a prime example of 'suffering for one's art'.

References

Altenmüller E: Robert Schumann's focal dystonia; in Bogousslavsky J, Boller F (eds): Neurological Disorders on Famous Artists. Front Neurol Neurosci. Basel, Karger, 2005, vol 19, pp 179–188.

Altenmüller E, Jabusch H-C: Musiker-Medizin; in Bruhn H, Kopiez R, Lehmann A (eds): Musikpsychologie. Das neue Handbuch. Reinbek, Rowohlt, 2008, pp 374–389.

Altenmüller E, McPherson G: Motor learning and instrumental training; in Gruhn W, Rauscher F (eds): Neurosciences in Music Pedagogy. New York, Nova Science, 2007, pp 121–144.

Brandfonbrener A, Kjelland J: Music medicine; in Parncutt R, McPherson G (eds): The Science and Psychology of Music Performance. New York, Oxford University Press, 2000, pp 83–96.

Czikszentmihalyi M: Flow: The Psychology of Optimal Experience. New York, Harper & Row, 1990.

De Vries C: Die Pianistin Clara Wieck-Schumann. Schumann Forschungen, vol. 5. Mainz, Schott, 1996.

Fields HL, Basbaum Al: Central nervous system mechanism of pain modulation; in Wall PD, Melzack R (eds): Textbook of Pain. Edinburgh, Churchill Livingstone, 1999, pp 309–329.

Fishbein M, Middlestadt S: Medical problems amongst ICSOM musicians. Overview of a national survey. Med Probl Perf Art 1988;3:1–8.

Flor H, Braun C, Elbert T, Birbaumer N: Extensive reorganization of primary somatosensory cortex in chronic back pain patients. Neurosci Lett 1997;224:5–8.

Gellrich M: Üben mit Lis(z)t. Frauenfeld, Waldgut, 1992, p 38.

Gerabek W, Haage BD, Keil G, Wegner W (eds): Enzyklopädie Medizingeschichte. Stuttgart, De Gruyter, 2005, p 1247.

Hammer M: Rheumatoide Arthritis; in Baron R, Strumpf M (eds): Praktische Schmerztherapie. Heidelberg, Springer, 2006, pp 265–267.

Klassen J: Clara Schumann: Musik und Öffentlichkeit. Cologne, Böhlau, 2009.

Köckritz C: Friedrich Wieck: Studien zur Biographie und zur Klavierpädagogik. Hildesheim, Olms Verlag, 2007.

Kopiez R, Lehmann AC, Klassen J: Clara Schumann's collection of playbills: a historiometric analysis of life-span development, mobility and repertoire canonization. Poetics 2009;37:50–73.

Litzmann B: Clara Schumann, Ein Künstlerleben. Nach Tagebüchern und Briefen, 3. Band. Leipzig, Breitkopf und Härtel, 1923.

Suaudeau C, Costentin J: Long lasting increase in nociceptive threshold induced in mice by forced swimming: involvement of an endorphinergic mechanism. Stress 2000;3:221–227.

Schumann R: Gesammelte Schriften, 1853, Wiesbaden, Neue Edition. Wiesbaden, VMA, 1962, p 234.

Shields N, Dockrell S: The prevalence of injuries among pianists in music schools in Ireland. Med Probl Perf Art 2000;15:155–167.

Steegmann M: Clara Schumann. RoRoRo-Monographien. Reinbeck, Rowohlt, 2001, p 14.

Tinazzi M, Fiaschi A, Rosso T, Faccioli F, Grosslercher J, Aglioti SM: Neuroplastic changes related to pain occur at multiple levels of the human somatosensory system: a somatosensory-evoked potentials study in patients with cervical radicular pain. J Neurosci 2000;20:9277–9283.

Walch-Schumann K (ed): Friedrich Wieck. Briefe aus den Jahren 1830–1838. Cologne, Arno Volk, 1968, p 39.

Wendler E: Clara Schumann: Das Band der ewigen Liebe. Briefwechsel mit Emilie und Elise List. Stuttgart, Metzler, 1996, p 137.

Univ. Prof. Dr. med. Eckart Altenmüller
Institut für Musikphysiologie und Musiker-Medizin
Hochschule für Musik und Theater Hannover
Hohenzollernstrasse 47
DE–30161 Hannover (Germany)
Tel. +49 0511 3100 552, Fax +49 0511 3100 557, E-Mail altenmueller@hmt-hannover.de

Bogousslavsky J, Hennerici MG, Bäzner H, Bassetti C (eds): Neurological Disorders in Famous Artists – Part 3. Front Neurol Neurosci. Basel, Karger, 2010, vol 27, pp 119–129

••••••••••••••••••••••

Bravo! Neurology at the Opera

Brandy R. Matthews

Indiana University School of Medicine, Indiana Alzheimer Disease Center,
Indianapolis, Ind., USA

Abstract

Opera is a complex musical form that reflects the complexity of the human condition and the human brain. This article presents an introduction to the portrayal of medical professionals in opera, including one neurologist, as well as two characters in whom neurological disease contributes to the action of the musical drama. Consideration is also given to the neuroanatomy and neuropathology of opera singers with further speculation regarding the neural underpinnings of the passion of opera's audience.

Copyright © 2010 S. Karger AG, Basel

The ability to create music is a universal human trait witnessed across societies throughout the ages. Song and dance continue to be pervasively used to tell stories of history and culture, to relax, and to simply entertain [Cross, 2003]. One such form of musical communication is opera, originating from the Latin for 'work' and sharing a root with the medical term 'operation' [http://www.merriam-webster.com/dictionary accessed Jan. 10, 2009]. Greenburg [1998] defines opera as 'a drama which combines soliloquy, dialogue, scenery, action, and continuous music with the whole to be greater than the parts'. With the advancement of neuroscience, it is increasingly more apparent that brain processes may actually contribute to this seemingly 'emergent property' of the opera experience.

The history of opera as a form of musical storytelling begins in the late Renaissance and early Baroque periods with composers such as Handel pursuing serious, often mythological, themes. As opera developed from the 18th through the 20th centuries, physicians and medical conditions began to be portrayed on the stage with variable prominence [Willich, 2006]. Herein brief consideration shall be given to the portrayal of physicians in opera, from *The Barber of Seville* to *Wozzeck*, culminating with an opera based on a neurologist's encounter with an interesting patient, *The Man Who Mistook His Wife for a Hat*. Additionally, two well-known operatic title characters suffering from presumed neurological disorders will be described, *Rigoletto* and Tom Rakewell of *The Rake's Progress*. In conclusion, a discussion of the neurology of vocal performance will be followed by what is currently known about the audience's oftentimes emotional response to operatic music.

Neurologists in Opera

In a systematic review of approximately 400 operas written in the 18th through 20th centuries, Willich [2006] identified 40 operas in which physicians appear on stage. The role of the physician in the action evolves in concordance with the social importance of physicians and the perception of medicine at the time the opera was conceived. Only one operatic character is clearly identified as a neurologist, but others provide context for the portrayal of both clinical and research medicine on stage. One of the early operatic physicians, Dr. Bartolo, a doctor in Gioacchino Rossini's *The Barber of Seville* [Rossini, 1816] provides a stark and unpleasant contrast to Figaro, a barber-surgeon, who offers the bulk of this opera's comedy and charm. Figaro, the jack-of-all-trades, assists in the deception of Dr. Bartolo, who is portrayed as arrogant and foolish as he plots to marry young Rosina for her inheritance. (It has been suggested in prior commentary on physicians in opera that Dr. Bartolo may not have been a medical doctor at all, but rather a doctor of law or some other area of study [Ober, 1976]; however, for purposes of this discussion we will assume that the composers and librettists were using the common connotation for the term.)

In Act I scene 1, Figaro celebrates his abilities by singing:

'Of a thousand professions, that of a barber is most noble…Razors, bibs, lancets and scissors, are always ready at my command…I am the city's factotum…Oh what a beautiful life! I tire little, and enjoy myself much…What a profession!' [Rossini, 1816, p 9].

On the contrary, in Act I scene 2, Dr. Bartolo is played a fool as he rests on his past accomplishments and perceived social role:

'To a doctor of my stature you dare offer such excuses…I advise you to use a better deception' [Rossini, 1816, p 35].

Although both characters portray a sense of inflated self-importance, the libretto and the score seem to support Figaro as the more likable character. With the evolution of medical practice, operas later in the 19th and 20th centuries tended to better acknowledge the role of a physician as a practitioner of medical science rather than simply a man with a title. However, even with its oversimplification of professional roles in medicine, this bel canto style comic opera may well have captured in exaggerated form a dichotomy between the so-called 'medical' and 'surgical' personalities which continues to fascinate modern audiences (i.e. the highly rated American television serials *House* and *Gray's Anatomy*).

A century later, the evolving role of physician as research scientist results in the sinister doctor of Alban Berg's 1922 opera Wozzeck [Goldovsky,1986]. Not specifically identified as a neurologist, this physician sacrifices the well-being of his patient in order to further his own prestige, captured in musical form by the use of dimunition, a technique in which faster note values of the same theme are repeated by the orchestra to emphasize the vocal pitch set [Florin, 2005]. In the heartless words of the doctor '…O, my theory, my fame! I shall be immortal! Immortal! Immortal! …' as Wozzeck, a poor soldier is increasingly delirious and eventually psychotic as a result of the doctor's experimentation [Berg, 1955]. The altered mental status could be a representation of the central nervous system manifestations of nutritional deficiencies related to thiamine, niacin, or cyanocobalamin, but the specific condition is of little importance to the drama in comparison to the ethics, or lack thereof, of the physician as researcher.

More recently, favorably combining the contemplative traits of the medical personality and the role of the physician as research scientist, composer Michael Nyman and librettist Christopher Rawlence have adapted neurologist Oliver Sacks' clinical tale 'The Man Who Mistook His Wife for a Hat' into a contemporary chamber opera. At last a neurologist takes center stage with such lyrical lines as,

'Neurology's favorite term is deficit. For all of these… we have private words of every sort: aphonia, aphemia, aphasia, alexia, apraxia, agnosia, amnesia, ataxia…' [Nyman,1987, p 45].

The action of the opera surrounds an accomplished musician who presents with his wife to a neurology clinic where little is initially revealed beyond a few visuo-perceptual mistakes. The neurologist makes a house call and discovers that the patient suffers from visual agnosia. The doctor also discovers that the patient copes with his perceptual impairment by relying on routines coupled with familiar music. The neurologist sings:

'He still has a perfect ear! His memory's unimpaired, perfect tonal and rhythmic discrimination and expression – but what of the parietal regions, the fibres, nerves, neurons, the synapses of the occipital zones? What of the cytoarchitectonic, the structure of visual processing? How? What? Does he see?' [Nyman, 1987, pp 83–85].

Thus, 'The Man Who Mistook His Wife for a Hat' is truly a neurologist's opera as it combines the portrayal of a physician clearly identified as a neurologist and his quest for neuroanatomic localization with a patient suffering from a complex neurological disease. Their series of clinical encounters highlight the importance of celebrating a patient's humanity no matter how unique or intel-

Table 1. Possible neurological causes of kypho-scoliosis in the title character of *Rigoletto*

Cerebral palsy	Duchenne muscular dystrophy
Neurofibromatosis type I	Spinal muscular atrophy
Syringomyelia	Pott disease (tuberculosis)
Fredreich ataxia	Poliomyelitis
Charcot-Marie-Tooth neuropathy	Klippel-Feil anomaly (with cervical cord compromise)

lectually stimulating 'the case' may be [St Louis, 1992]. Moreover, this story remains especially timely as the patient on whom the title character was based most likely suffered from an atypical form of Alzheimer's disease [Sacks, 2007], one of the most prevalent neurological disorders in the world [Qiu et al, 2009].

Neurological Disease in Opera

Like the visual agnosia clearly identified and pivotal to the action of 'The Man Who Mistook His Wife for a Hat', the portrayal of an entirely different neuro-orthopedic condition [Fardon, 2002] plays a central role in the development of the action in Verdi's *Rigoletto* [1851]. The title character, a court jester, is portrayed as predominantly sympathetic, but inevitably cursed in the context of his physical deformity, a so-called 'hunchback', to which he solemnly refers:

'Oh rabbia! Esser difforme!' (Oh what a fate! To be deformed!) [Verdi, 1851, p 17].

His kypho-scoliosis may have resulted from any number of disorders, ranging from congenital anomalies to trauma, but according to a well-respected pediatric neurology textbook, 'The presence of scoliosis... in males of all ages should strongly suggest either a spinal cord disorder or a neuromuscular disease' [Fenichel, 1997]. Bearing this modern diagnostic pearl in mind, considerations in the differential diagnosis of Rigoletto include congenital and neurogenetic disorders as well as neuroinfectious etiologies (table 1).

While further diagnostic clues are seemingly absent from the libretto, it is clear that the courtiers are disgusted by Rigoletto's outward appearance when, after mistaking his daughter for his mistress, they comment with surprise,

'Perduto ha la gobba? Non e piu difforme?' (Has he lost his hunchback? He's no longer deformed?) [Verdi, 1851, p 7].

As is the case in all tragic operas, Rigoletto cannot escape his curse, and loses all that he loves in the end. This may reflect the pervasive attitude of the time toward patients struck with disfiguring conditions, a mixture of sympathy and an irrational fear of contagion and 'bad luck'.

In a less transparent example, *The Rake's Progress* most likely portrays dementia paralytica associated with neurosyphilis. Igor Stravinsky's only full-length opera paired with W.H. Auden and Chester Kallman's libretto is loosely based on the engravings of William Hogarth. The opera, originally produced in 1951, portrays the title character, Tom Rakewell, departing from his beloved and descending into a world of gambling, fornication, and risky investments, eventually losing his entire fortune in addition to his sanity. The power of Tom's love saves him from suicide, but he is cursed with 'madness' as a consequence of his reckless behavior. While there is no direct reference to venereal disease in the opera, musical reference to cause and effect as well as the historical context of the opera suggest that spirochete infection results in Rakewell's progressive and persistent dementia. Most notably, a similar chorus in the key of C appears only in the brothel and Bedlam scenes (fig. 1, 2), suggesting that the locations are one in the same, or one the result of the other [Hutcheon and Hutcheon, 1996]. Epidemiology provides an equally important clue to the neurological disease portrayed on stage, as the prevalence of syphilis at the time of the opera's debut was markedly higher at around 65 per 100,000 population in the 1940s compared to approximately 2.5 per 100,000 population in 2004 [Kent and Romanelli, 2008]. With the accessibility of screening tests of the serum and CSF, and intramuscular and intravenous antibiotics, the incidence of tertiary syphilis and its associated frontal and temporal lobe predominant dementia paralytica has plummeted. However, the themes of *The Rake's Progress* remain timely as other communicable diseases such as HIV have potentially delayed, yet equally devastating, neuropsychiatric consequences [Dubé et al., 2005].

Neurology of Vocal Performance

Vocal artistry most commonly predominated over orchestration and staging in opera performance of the 18th, 19th, and much of the 20th centuries. The neuroanatomy of singing is complex and involves all of the component parts of motor speech, including: respiration, phonation, resonation, and articulation. Respiration is supported by the diaphragm innervated by C3–5 nerve roots as well as the intercostal and abdominal musculature. Phonation and resonation involve the 9th and 10th cranial nerves, and articulation is reliant upon cranial nerves 7 and 12. The activity of the vocal folds is dependent on the function of the recurrent and superior laryngeal divisions of the vagus nerve. During

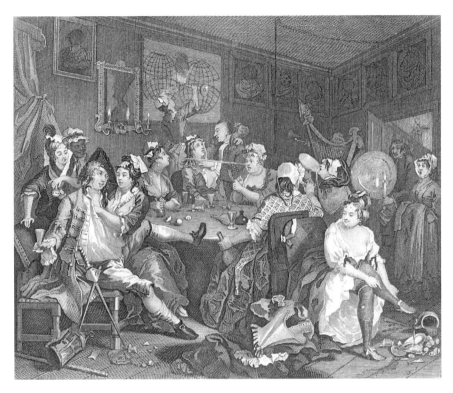

Fig. 1. The Rake's Progress Plate 3: Tavern Scene. Engraver: William Hogarth, in The Works of William Hogarth. In a series of engravings with descriptions, and a comment on their moral tendency by John Trusler (contributors John Hogarth and John Nichols). Original publication London, Jones, 1833. Current release date: Sept 4, 2007 [EBook No. 22500]. http://www.gutenberg.org/files/22500/22500-h/22500-h.htm. Accessed Oct 15, 2009.

phonation, the vocal folds are brought together near the center of the larynx by muscles attached to the arytenoids (fig. 3). As air is forced through the vocal folds, they vibrate and produce sound. By contracting or relaxing the muscles of the arytenoids, the qualities of this sound can be altered.

Additional neuroanatomic contributions to voice include circuits representing cortical motor control areas for the larynx and articulators as well as subcortical and cerebellar implicit motor memory areas. Vocal training increases activation on functional MRI scans in areas including the primary somatosensory cortex for vocalization, which demonstrates a greater activation in the right hemisphere in professional opera singers. Expert singers also

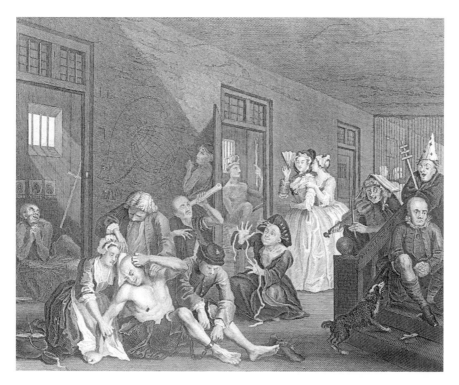

Fig. 2. The Rake's Progress Plate 8: Scene in Bedlam. Engraver: William Hogarth, in The Works of William Hogarth. In a series of engravings with descriptions, and a comment on their moral tendency by John Trusler (contributors John Hogarth and John Nichols). Original publication London, Jones, 1833. Current release date: Sept 4, 2007 [EBook No. 22500]. http://www.gutenberg.org/files/22500/22500-h/22500-h.htm. Accessed Oct 15, 2009.

demonstrate increased activation in the thalamus, basal ganglia, and cerebellum [Kleber et al., 2009]. Comparing professional vocalists with 'tone-deaf' singers suggests that a lack of connections between auditory and motor regions may result in poor vocal ability while the duration of vocal training for professional singers may correlate with both gray and white matter 'enhancements' [Schlaug, 2009].

Neurological disorders are not restricted to opera characters; the opera performers may also be afflicted with neurological disease from stage fright with dysautonomia to recurrent laryngeal nerve damage subsequent to chest surgery [Gould, 1986]. Also described is singer's dystonia which, like vocal dystonia that affects conversational speech, may have either an adductor or abductor

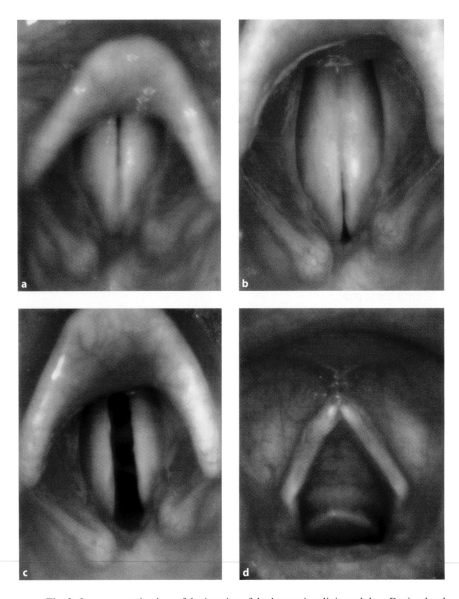

Fig. 3. Laryngoscopic view of the interior of the larynx in a living adult. *a* During loud phonation. *b* During whispering. *c* During quiet respiration. *d* During forced inspiration. From Köpf-Maier [2005].

character. Similar to other task-specific musicians' dystonias and overuse syndromes [Lockwood, 1989], singer's dystonia can be disabling from a vocational perspective given the associated loss of vibrato and truncated range observed in those afflicted [Chitkara et al., 2006].

Neurology of Opera's Audience

The portrayal of physicians (and a single neurologist) and neurological disease have obviously had a relatively minimal impact on the history of opera while the neuroanatomy of vocal performance has decidedly helped shaped the art form. Nevertheless, audience neurology, and the emotional response to opera in particular, may be the most important contributor to the perpetuation of opera performance, as the contemporary lack of widespread social and financial support for the art form cannot diminish the passion of opera fans [Stone, 2009]. While it is possible that opera fans are simply more passionate individuals, with some published evidence that opera fans are more likely than non-fans to accept suicide in the context of dishonor [Stack, 2002], it is equally tenable that it is primarily the emotional experience of perceiving live opera that compels a patron to return. The physicality of this experience from a fan perspective is well captured by Flaubert in *Madame Bovary* as Emma Bovary attends a performance of Donizetti's *Lucia di Lammermoor:*

'She yielded to the rippling of the melodies and she felt herself trembling all over, as though the bows of the violins were being drawn across her nerves.' [Flaubert, 1857, p 206].

Neuroscience has only recently begun to tackle the challenge of understanding such a profoundly emotional response to music. This response appears to vary according to musical training, be related to specific musical variables including tempo and mode, and may be mediated by subcortical dopaminergic pleasure circuits or even opioid receptors in the brainstem [Matthews, 2008]. It has even been hypothesized that the human mirror neuron system plays a role in the structural analysis of music, following auditory signal processing in the superior temporal gyrus and preceding emotional awareness and response processing in the anterior insula and limbic system [Molnar-Szakacs and Overy, 2006].

Opera extends beyond the labyrinthine human emotional response to music with the addition of language, an equally complicated stimulus. Functional MRI and electrophysiological data reveal an overlapping brain network of frontal and temporal regions responsible for the processing of songs with lyrics in which each dimension (language vs. music) is influenced by the processing of the other in an elaborate interaction [Schon et al., 2005]. Furthermore, as noted by Hutcheon and Hutcheon [2000] in *Bodily Charm: Living Opera*, the emotional response to opera is not merely a response to music and language, but to the elements of comedy or drama with all of the other multi-modal sensory stimuli from elaborate sets to the responses of other audience members. Again, Flaubert captures the depth of this experience with Emma Bovary's trip to the opera:

'Two eyes were not enough to take in the costumes, the scenery, the characters…the velvet caps, the cloaks, the swords, that whole imaginary world pulsing to the music as though in the atmosphere of some other realm' [Flaubert, 1857, pp 206–207].

It seems as though the experience of opera may exceed the current framework of neuroscientific reductionism; thankfully this does not detract from the pleasure to be derived by those enchanted with both.

References

Berg A: Georg Buchner's Wozzeck: Opera in 3 Acts (15 scenes). Translated by Blackhall E, Harford V. Vienna, Universal Edition, 1955.
Chitkara A, Meyer T, Keidar A, Blitzer A: Singer's dystonia: first report of a variant of spasmodic dysphonia. Ann Otol Rhinol Laryngol 2006;115:89–92.
Cross I: Music as a biocultural phenomenon. Ann NY Acad Sci 2003;999:106–111.
Dubé B, Benton T, Cruess DG, Evans DL: Neuropsychiatric manifestations of HIV infection and AIDS. J Psychiatry Neurosci 2005;30:237–246.
Fardon D: Spine in the arts: the hunchback of the opera. Spine J 2002;2:158.
Fenichel GM: Clinical Pediatric Neurology. ed 3. Philadelphia, Saunders,1997, p 258.
Flaubert G: Madame Bovary. orig. 1857. Translated by Wall G. London, Penguin, 1992, pp 206–207.
Florin TA: Demon, quack, scientist, or saint. Depictions of doctoring in the operatic literature. Pharos Alpha Omega Alpha Honro Med Soc 2005;6818–6824.
Goldovsky B: Some medical matters in operatic literature. Cleve Clin Q 1986;53:39–43.
Gould WJ: Some specific problems of professional operatic singers. Cleve Clin Q 1986;53:45–47.
Greenberg R: How to Listen to and Understand Opera, Part I, Lecture 1. The Teaching Company Course No. 740. Chantilly, Teaching Company Limited Partnership, 1998.
Hutcheon M, Hutcheon L: The Perceiving Body; in Bodily Charm: Living Opera. Lincoln, University of Nebraska Press, 2000, p156.
Hutcheon M, Hutcheon L: The Pox Revisited: The Pale Spirochete; in Twentieth Century Opera in Opera: Desire, Disease, Death. Lincoln, University of Nebraska Press, 1996, pp 95–117.
Kent ME, Romanelli F: Re-examining syphilis: an update on epidemiology, clinical manifestations, and management. Ann Pharmacother 2008;42:226–236.
Kleber B, Veit R, Birbaumer N, Gruzelier J, Lotze M: The brain of opera singers: experience-dependent changes in functional activation. Cerebral Cortex 2009, epub ahead of print.
Köpf-Maier P: Wolf-Heidegger's Atlas of Human Anatomy, ed 6. Basel, Karger, 2005, vol 2.
Lockwood AH: Medical problems of musicians. N Engl J Med 1989;320:221–227.
Matthews B: The musical brain; in Goldenberg G, Miller BL (eds): The Handbook of Clinical Neurology, 3rd ser: Neuropsychology and Behavioral Neurology. London, Elsevier, 2008, vol 88, pp 464–466.
Molnar-Szakacs I, Overy K: Music and mirror neurons: from motion to 'e'motion. Soc Cogn Affect Neurosci 2006;1:235–241.
Nyman M: The Man Who Mistook his Wife for a Hat. Based on story by Sacks O with libretto by Rawlence C. CBS Masterworks 44669 booklet notes, 1987.

Ober W: Operatic 'doctors'. Practitioner 1976;216:110–116.

Qiu C, Kivipelto M, von Strauss E: Epidemiology of Alzheimer's disease: occurrence, determinants, and strategies toward intervention. Dialogues Clin Neurosci 2009;11:111–128.

Rossini G: Il barbiere di Siviglia. Based on story by Beaumarchais with libretto by Sterbini C. Orig. 1816. Libretto translator Fisher B. Opera Journeys Publishing Trans 2001 (rev. 2007).

Sacks O: Musicophilia. New York, Knopf, 2007, p 236.

Schlaug, G: Singing in the brain: professional singers, occasional singers, and out-of-tune singers. J Acoust Soc Am 2009;126:2277.

Schon D, Gordon RL, Besson M: Musical and linguistic processing in song perception. Ann NY Acad Sci 2005;1060:71–81.

St Louis EK: The physician in contemporary opera: three divergent approaches to the doctor-patient relationship. Pharos Alpha Omega Alpha Honor Med Soc 1992;55:15–20.

Stack S: Opera subculture and suicide for honor. Death Stud 2002;26:431–437.

Stone A: Fine arts are in survival mode as funds dry up. USA Today online version Feb 3, 2009 http://www.usatoday.com/life/theater/2009-03-01-artseconomy_N.html accessed Oct 15, 2009.

Verdi G: Rigoletto: An Opera in Four Acts. Based on story by Hugo V with libretto by Piave F. Orig. 1851. Libretto translator Fisher B. Opera Journeys Publishing Trans 2001 (rev. 2005).

Willich SN: The physician as opera character: a reflection of medical history and public perception. BMJ 2006;333:1333–1335.

Brandy R. Matthews, MD
Indiana University Neurology Outpatient Clinic
550 University Blvd UH 1710
Indianapolis, IN 46202 (USA)
Tel. +1 317 944 4000, Fax +1 317 278 2775, E-Mail brmatthe@iupui.edu

Bogousslavsky J, Hennerici MG, Bäzner H, Bassetti C (eds): Neurological Disorders in Famous Artists – Part 3. Front Neurol Neurosci. Basel, Karger, 2010, vol 27, pp 130–142

....

Stendhal's Aphasic Spells: The First Report of Transient Ischemic Attacks Followed by Stroke

Julien Bogousslavsky[a], *Gil Assal*[b]

[a]Center for Brain and Nervous System Disorders, and Neurorehabilitation Services, Genolier Swiss Medical Network, Clinique Valmont, Montreux, and [b]Lausanne, Switzerland

Abstract

In March 1841, the year before he died of acute stroke, Stendhal, one of the most famous French novelists of the 19th century, developed a series of short-lived speech impairments which he precisely reported in his correspondence. His reports suggest that these spells were aphasic transient ischemic attacks (TIAs). The accuracy and precision of Stendhal's description exactly 20 years before Broca's presentation at the Société d'Anthropologie is remarkable since it occurred at a time when TIAs had not been studied in the medical literature and aphasia was still in its 'prehistory'. Stendhal's TIAs a few months before his fatal stroke constitute the first historical report of the warning nature of TIAs, which would be emphasized only over 100 years later.

Henri-Marie Beyle was born in Grenoble, France, in 1783, and he died 59 years later in Paris from what was then called apoplexy. He made a military and diplomatic career, being appointed 'consul de France' for the Austrian States in Trieste in 1830, and later in Civita-Vecchia (Roman States). However, he is better known as *Stendhal*, one of the major French novelists of the 19th century ('La Chartreuse de Parme', 'Le Rouge et le Noir'). He took this pseudonym for his 3rd book 'Rome, Naples et Florence' in 1817, adding an 'h' to the name of the small Prussian town Stendal, where the famous art historian Johann Winckelmann came from. He thought that taking a name with Germanic features would be helpful to support his virulent writing against the state in which Italy had been left after the Congress of Vienna.

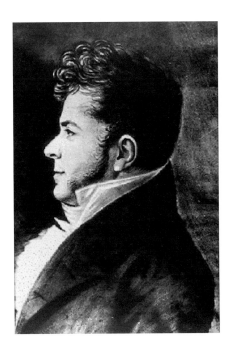

Fig. 1. Stendhal as a young man, by Quenedey.

Stendhal was a very lively, emotional, character, who was frequently involved in complicated affairs with women of very different origins. He was slightly fat (fig. 1), and it seems that certain of his medical problems, such as gout or chest pain, were commonly triggered by affective changes in his life. For instance, in 1818, after his break up with Angela Pietragrua, 'this sublime whore', his health declined, and he drew a diagram which emphasized a progressive increase in 'angina pectoris' [Del Litto, 1968]. However, it was only over 20 years later that Stendhal developed the first manifestations of the disease which finally killed him.

Stendhal and Medicine

Stendhal did not have a very good opinion of medicine and physicians [Ansel et al., 2003], as will be exemplified below when he developed warning transient aphasic episodes one year before he died of a stroke. In his novels, there are few precise diseases, contrary to a much higher frequency of violent wounds. The heroes typically die at a rather young age ('a good hero is a dead hero'), while doctors usually are depicted as grotesque figures or intrigants.

More than in somatic medicine, Stendhal was interested in the emerging psychiatry. He often referred to 'folly', usually underlining its positive and creative aspects [Felman, 1971]. Memory was also of interest to him: he defined it as 'the power through which an image or a concept remains in the head'. He frequently quoted his own 'memory holes', and he said that he could not remember entire periods of his life. He even used these lacunas in certain autobiographic writings to purposefully give the manuscript a discontinued or unfinished color. Stendhal read and admired two physicians who were involved in mental disorders in his time. The first was Pierre Jean Georges Cabanis (1757–1808) who was a professor of hygiene and clinical medicine and had helped Bonaparte to take power; Stendhal especially liked his theory of tempers and instincts which he used in his novels. Philippe Pinel (1745–1828), from La Salpêtrière, was the second. He was what one called at that time an 'alienist', and had largely contributed to the renewal of ideas and management in mental medicine. In 1806, Stendhal read his famous 'Traité médico-philosophique sur l'aliénation mentale, ou la manie' [Pinel, 1802], which he strongly advised his sister Pauline to read.

Much later, Stendhal was indirectly associated with a psychiatric syndrome, now know as 'Stendhal syndrome' [Magherini, 1989], also called Florence syndrome, which corresponds to a feeling of self-disintegration and mental decay associated with an overflow of cultural or esthetic emotional stimuli (also enlarged to include love). This referred to Stendhal's experience which he reported and used for his second book 'Histoire de la peinture en Italie' (1817) which, for the first time, contains the famous 'To the happy few': 'The Sybils of Volterrano gave me the most precious delight I have ever derived from painting (…) I was dead tired with swollen feet, aching in narrow shoes; although a petty sensation it still would have prevented me from admiring God in all his glory – but in front of this picture I totally forgot it. My heavens, how beautiful it is! (…) I got into the state of emotion where the "celestial sensations" of the fine arts encounter impassionated sentiments. When leaving Santa Croce, I had heart palpitations, what one calls "nerves" in Berlin; life was exhausted in me, I was walking in fear of falling down'. This extraordinary experience was also reinforced by Bronzino's 'The Descent of Christ into Limbo'.

Another intriguing phenomenon was reported by Stendhal [Ansel et al., 2003] who found that good odors triggered 'weakening in my left arm and leg and give me the feeling of falling on that side'. Since Stendhal complained of repeated headaches (which he himself called migraine) most of his life, one may wonder whether this could have been a migrainous phenomenon. Years later, when Stendhal had his aphasic spells, he attributed them either to gout or migraine. However, it is unfortunate that descriptions of Stendhal's 'migraines' and possible neurologic accompaniments are lacking.

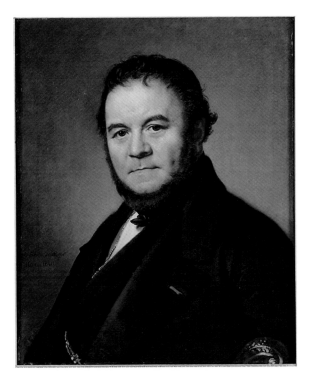

Fig. 2. Stendhal by Soedermark, 1840, a few years before his TIAs and stroke. Musée National du Château de Versailles. ©Photo RMN, with kind permission.

Stendhal's Aphasic Transient Ischemic Attacks and Final Stroke

Stendhal died of a stroke which was preceded several months before by TIAs and manifested as impaired speech (fig. 2). Despite the importance of these events in Stendhal's life, as well as the important issue of the loss of language in a famous writer, it is striking that Stendhal's illness was emphasized very little, a good example being the absence of reference to stroke, apoplexy, brain attack or aphasia in the 'Dictionnaire de Stendhal' (Stendhal dictionary), published in 2003 [Ansel et al., 2003].

One year before his death, on March 15, 1841, he had several spells of speech loss which he described very precisely in letters to his friends. Around one year earlier, on January 1, 1840, he experienced a spell of another type while he working on his book 'Lamiel': a sudden dizziness made him fall into the burning fireplace. On April 5, 1841, he wrote to Domenico Fiore (1769–1848), a dear friend whom he had met in 1821 and who largely contributed to his nomination as 'consul': '(…) horrible migraines for six months; then, four spells of the following sickness: All of a sudden I forget all French words. I can no longer say: "Give me a glass of water". I watch myself with curiosity; apart from the ability to use words, I keep all the natural properties of "the animal". It lasts eight to ten minutes; then, slowly, the memory of words comes back, and I am tired (…) I had four suppressions of any memory of all French language; it lasts six to eight minutes; ideas are fine, but without words. Ten days ago, while dining at the cabaret with Constantin, I made incredible efforts to find the word "glass". I still have some background headache, coming from the stomach, and I am tired from having tried to write these three pages not too badly. During the spell before the last one, in the early morning, I continued to dress to go hunting; the better to stay quiet here than in any other place. "Vale"' [Stendhal, 1968]. In that letter, Stendhal also mentions that a homeopath from Berlin told him that this was some kind of 'nervous apoplexy'. He added that he plans to obtain a consultation with Pierre Prévost in Geneva, who already cured his gout, although he 'believes little in medicine, especially in doctors, mediocre men'. The homeopath, with a 'naughty, spiritual physiognomy' and a 'crook speech', gave him aconite 'to animate circulation', and prescribed sulfur. Apparently another spell occurred at another time, on April 9, and the next day Stendhal wrote to Fiore that 'this unpleasant phenomenon recurred', which he called 'thick tongue'. He also complained of transient suffocations, which made him believe that he would die, and wondered whether homeopathy may also make one die from apoplexy. On April 19, he wrote again to Fiore that 'the most unpleasant symptom is the awkwardness of the tongue, which makes me stutter'. A later post-scriptum adds: 'On April 20, attack of weakness in the left leg and thigh. Alright on April 21'. While it has been suggested that his last portrait, by Henry Lehmann (in August 1841; fig. 3), shows signs of right face and hand weakness [Del Litto, 1968], a close examination of that portrait is not conclusive, and Stendhal indeed never reported right hemiparesis as one would have expected in association with aphasia. The meaning of the left-side involvement in the lower limb on April 21 remains unknown since Stendhal was clearly right-handed, and we have no clue against a usual language lateralization in the left hemisphere. The possibility of non-simultaneous TIAs in both hemispheres cannot be discarded, and would suggest either bilateral internal carotid artery disease or a cardio-embolic source. Apparently, no further episodes occurred. Stendhal had several treatments including venous taps and, among several doctors, was seen by the Pope's physician Dr. Alertz from Aix-la-Chapelle.

While the spells of speech loss were reported by Stendhal to have been short-lived, it is not impossible that the first ones led to longer-lasting language impairment as suggested by the first note dated March 15 in his diary [Stendhal, 1982]: 'Je vois le professeur Dalbret qui est d'avis de goutte voulant venir à la

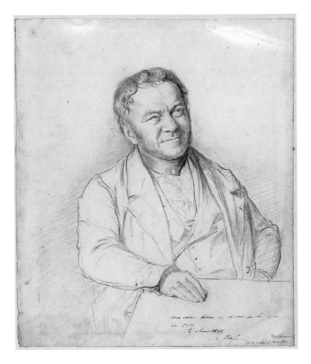

Fig. 3. Stendhal last portrait, by Henry Lehmann, August 1841. Musée Stendhal, Grenoble, No. 836, with kind permission.

tête', which is quite linguistically incorrect for a professional writer, and totally unusual under Stendhal's pen. Unfortunately, very little was added by Stendhal in his diary, and on March 16, he just mentioned: 'the tongue on the 14th and 15th'. However, no language dysfunction can be seen in the five letters he wrote between March 15 and his first letter to Fiore about the spells [Stendhal, 1968]. The first letter after March 15 is dated March 21, to Jean-Victor Schnetz, who was the successor to Ingres as the director of the 'Académie de France' in Rome. Stendhal only mentioned that he 'underwent a venous tap in the morning because an infamous migraine'. Then, he wrote three letters to François Guizot, the Minister of Foreign Affairs of Louis-Philippe in France, and one to his fellow novelist Honoré de Balzac, without mentioning any health problem and with normal writing and content.

Apparently, Stendhal rapidly recovered as from early August he was involved in a slightly complicated affair with the daughter of a famous singer, Cecchina Lablache, who seemingly omitted to inform Stendhal of the pres-

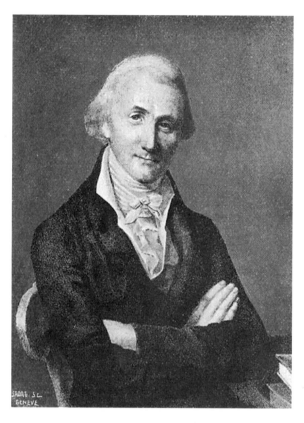

Fig. 4. Dr. Pierre Prévost, from Geneva, whom Stendhal consulted shortly after his aphasic TIAs. Courtesy Olivier Walusinski Library, Brou, France.

ence of a husband and another lover. On August 9, he summarized his disease to Guizot, writing that 'gout had been threatening with a brain congestion'. He saw Dr. Prévost (fig. 4) in Geneva between the end of October and the beginning of November. The impression of the physician was not good, and new 'malaises' delayed a trip to Paris. On November 8, his cousin and friend Romain Colomb found that Stendhal's conversation was slower and less subtle than before [Colomb, 1854]. On March 22, 1842, Stendhal wrote in his diary that he had written 15 pages of a manuscript the day before [Stendhal, 1982]. But at 7 p.m., in the rue Neuve-des-Capucines (today the part of rue des Capucines closest to the boulevard), perhaps just when leaving the Ministery of Foreign Affairs building, Stendhal fell heavily on the sidewalk. Colomb was there 20 minutes later and found his cousin unconscious and without any reactions. He was given first care without success by Dr. Eyland and Dr. Prus, who were nearby. Stendhal was transported to a small shop nearby and then to the 'Hôtel de Nantes', where he was staying, at 78 rue Neuve-des-Petits-Champs, which was an elongation of the street where he had fallen [Doyon, 1966, 1967]. Colomb [1854] wrote: '(…) he expired on Wednesday, March 23, 1842, at 2 a.m., with no suffering, without having uttered a single word, and at the age of fifty-nine years, one month and twenty-eight days'. No mention of hemiplegia or any other focal brain dysfunction was mentioned, but the diagnosis was apoplexy, which Colomb attributed to the fact that during the preceding eight days, Stendhal had resumed literary activities against the recommendation of his doctor. No autopsy was performed and, the day after his death, Stendhal was buried in the Montmartre cemetery. The immediate severity of the stroke suggests a massive brain hemorrhage or infarction, but its vascular territory remains unknown, as is the potential relationship between the TIAs of 1841 and the lethal stroke. Stendhal was struck while walking in the street, so that what he had written to Fiore on April 10, 1841, shortly after his TIAs, sounds strangely premonitory [Stendhal, 1968]: 'I find that it is not ridiculous to die in the street, when not on purpose.'

Early Reports of TIAs

It is the custom to attribute the first description of a TIA to William Heberden (1710–1801) in his 1802 posthumous book: 'A numbness of the hand may come on first day, on the second a faltering voice and on the third a palsy' [Fields, 1998]. However, this description rather suggests a progressing or fluctuating stroke. In fact, a description and a concept of TIAs are hard to find in the medical literature of the 19th century and the first half of the 20th century. The issue of circulatory 'insufficiency' was based on the emphasis of hemodynamic failure as a common cause of focal brain ischemia, which was subsequently found to be quite rare [Paciaroni and Bogousslavsky, 2009]. It was only several decades later that Charles Miller Fisher introduced the term 'intermittent cerebral ischemia' in 1958 [Fisher, 1958], followed by 'transient ischemic attack', the use of which became wide only after the 4th Princeton Conference in 1965 [Carolei et al., 1998]. Initially, the TIA duration was rightly limited to less than 1 h, before it was extended to 24 h in classifications. We now know that most TIAs last much less than 1 h, and usually do not extend beyond the 10 min mentioned by Stendhal in his letter to Fiore. In fact, most so-called 'TIAs' lasting more than 1 h correspond to 'cerebral infarcts with transient signs' (CITS), because a longer duration is associated with permanent ischemic brain damage [Bogousslavsky and Regli, 1984]. The acceptance of the term 'TIA' occurred in parallel to the demonstration that these events are usually of an embolic – not hemodynamic –nature, a fact which had already been evoked, and was subsequently well established, for cerebral infarcts (Wepfer, Bayle, Virchow, Gowers, Gull, Ramsay Hunt), either from a cardiac or an arterial source [Paciaroni and Bogousslavsky, 2009]. The interest of the TIA concept was its identification as a warning sign announcing a high risk of brain infarction with permanent neurologic damage [Carolei et al., 1998]. We do not know whether Stendhal's TIAs in 1841 could have been regarded as directly 'announcing' his fatal stroke in 1842, since we know so little about that stroke, but they probably are the first accurate report of focal TIAs followed by stroke, emphasizing the warning nature of the former.

Early Reports of Aphasia

In 1745, the naturalist Carolus Linnaeus [1707–1778] mentioned the possibility of a language disorder consisting in knowing what one wishes to say without being able to say it, without altered oral or written comprehension [Viets, 1943]. Shortly thereafter, von Swieten also reported that he had seen several patients who 'would try with their hands and feet and their whole body to explain what they wanted and yet could not' [von Swieten, 1754]. A century before, Thomas Willis and some of his contemporaries already reported cases which would now be qualified as aphasic [Fields and Lemak, 1989]. Much earlier, while loss of speech seems to have been mentioned from the time of Aristotle, no detail was usually given, and the typical explanation was of an awkwardness of the tongue [Critchley, 1970]. Macdonald Critchley, in an essay on aphasiology [1970], quoted the self-reported case of Spalding in 1772, which appears to be the first accurate description of a transient speech disorder, in fact very similar to what Stendhal himself reported: 'Under the impact of those wavy and entangled images I tried to catch basic tenets of religion, conscience, and expectation of future salvation (…) I could not get the better of that crowding and that stir and bustle in my head. I tried to speak, to train myself as it were, and to test whether I could say something in a connected order; but much as I forced my attention and my thoughts and proceeded with the utmost slowness, I became aware very soon of monstrous shapeless words that were absolutely different from those I intended; my immortal soul was at present as little master of the inner tools of language as it has been before of my writing.' It seems that after half an hour, Spalding's speech began to recover: 'Those strange annoying ideas (and images) became less lively and buzzing. I was able to get through what I wanted to think, and the interruptions by those strange ideas became weaker.' But perhaps the most famous early description of aphasia is the self-report by Samuel Johnson (1709–1784), then aged 73 years (by the way, also suspected to have suffered from Gilles de la Tourette's disease), in a series of letter to friends accounting for what happened to him on June 17, 1783, for about one week, 18 months before his death from cardiopulmonary failure. These letters have been detailed elsewhere [Critchley, 1970], and the most famous anecdote of this episode is the attempt of Johnson to repeat the Lord's Prayer in Latin, while he observed that he had lost the words in English. While the letters (the first letter to Edmund Allen being already dated from the first day) disclose a few agraphic features, a rather selective impairment of oral language without hand palsy allowed this fascinating self-report: 'It has pleased almighty God this morning to deprive me of the powers of speech'… William Heberden himself examined Johnson whose aphasia seems to have nearly recovered within less than 10 days. It is ironic that 35 years later, and 25 years before losing his speech abilities himself, Stendhal would plagiarize Johnson's preface to Shakespeare's works in the first chapter of an essay on 'Qu'est-ce que le romanticisme' (a play of words mixing romanticism with 'roman', which in French means a 'novel') [Ansel et al., 2003].

However, the first modern description and study of a case of aphasia is another self-report, the one by Jacques Lordat (1773–1870; fig. 5) following a stroke (at age 52) due to the now very uncommon cause of a tonsil abscess which likely led to in situ thrombosis of the carotid artery [Ombredane, 1951; Hécaen and Dubois, 1969]. Lordat was a doctor, and this probably allowed him to report in detail that particular event (which had taken place in July 1825) during his physiology course in 1842–1843 at Montpellier, where he had been appointed professor of anatomy and physiology in 1813. He called it 'verbal amnesia', also using the term 'alalia', which had been proposed by Delius in 1757, and which Lordat had already used in 1820 [Bayle, 1939]. He did not make any anatomical-clinical reference, but elaborated a theory on the ten acts which lead from thought to sound emission. Lordat defined alalia as a disorder of the material transformation of ideas into sounds, corresponding to impaired remembering of previous sounds stored into memory, together with a dysfunction of the syntactic organization of sounds (Lordat 1843). He also insisted on the integrity of his intelligence and the preservation of his inner thinking when he was alone while unable to speak, and did not need to speak. Lordat recovered fully and died at 97, 45 years after his stroke, having resumed all his activities. The same year as Lordat's stroke, Jean-Baptiste Bouillaud (1796–1881), who later became the model for Dr. Horace Bianchon in Balzac's 'La Comédie Humaine' ('La Cousine Bette'), published his treatise on encephalitis, in which a first attempt to localize speech in the brain was made from a scientific point of view [Bouillaud, 1825]: Bouillaud underlined the role of the frontal regions more than 35 years before Broca, but he missed the fact that most of his obser-

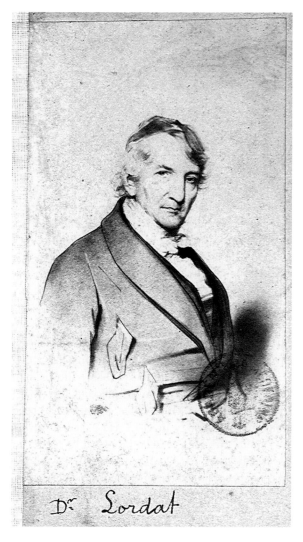

Fig. 5. Dr. Jacques Lordat, from Montpellier, who made the first detailed self-report and study on aphasia. Courtesy Olivier Walusinski Library, Brou, France.

vations pointed to a lateralized lesion in the left hemisphere. Ten years later at the 1836 Congrès Méridional de Montpellier, this fact did not escape the general practitioner from Sommières, Marc Dax (1771–1837), when he emphasized that 'lesions of the left half of the brain correspond to the forgetting of thought signs'. Dax based his claim on two cases he had seen in 1800 and 1809, plus the case of Pierre Broussonnet (a naturalist from Montpellier and a university colleague of Lordat, whose obituary was written by Baron Cuvier and Augustin de Candolle) [Héral, 2009]. However, since there were no published proceedings of the Montpellier congress, Dax's observations were made public by his son Gustave in 1863 (and published in 1865), but only after Broca's report in 1861.

However, at the time of Stendhal's TIAs and stroke, the phrenology of F.J. Gall was still a successful leading theory among scientists. Franz Josef Gallo, better known as F.J. Gall (1758–1828), was really the first anatomist to focus on the correlation of higher mental functions within the cerebral cortex, and he mentioned cases of aphasia, including one of a wound in the frontal region. Bouillaud was greatly influenced by Gall's work, which inspired his emphasis on the involvement of the anterior lobules in the loss of ability to evoke words and combine them into sentences [Hécaen and Lanteri-Laura, 1978]. It is a striking coincidence that in October 1841, exactly when Stendhal was seeking the advice of Prévost for his intermittent speech disturbances, Paul Broca (1824–1880), then aged 17 years, took the carriage from Bordeaux to Paris to study medicine [Schiller, 1979], just 20 years before he made the famous presentation of the case of Leborgne at the Société d'Anthropologie, which would put an end to what can be called the prehistory of aphasia.

Thus it is particularly striking that at a time when neither aphasia nor TIAs were well described and studied in the medical literature, one of the most famous French novelists so precisely reported his own experience of aphasic TIAs, before his own death from stroke provided the first historical confirmation of the warning nature of TIAs.

References

Ansel Y, Berthier P, Nerlich M: Dictionnaire de Stendhal. Paris, Honoré Champion, 2003.

Bayle MJM: Les fondateurs de la doctrine française de l'aphasie; thèse. Bordeaux, Imprimerie de Bière, 1939.

Bogousslavsky J, Regli F: Cerebral infarction with transient signs (CITS): do TIAs correspond to small deep infarcts in internal carotid artery occlusion? Stroke 1984;15:536–539.

Bouillaud MJ: Traité clinique et physiologique de l'encéphalite ou inflammation du cerveau et de ses suites. Paris, Baillière, 1825.

Carolei A, Marini C, Fieschi C: Transient ischemic attacks; in Ginsberg MD, Bogousslavsky J (eds): Cerebrovascular Disease, Pathophysiology, Diagnosis, and Management. New York, Blackwell Science, 1998, pp 941–960.

Colomb R: Notice sur la vie et les ouvrages de M. Beyle Stendhal. Paris, Imprimerie Vve Dondey Dupré, 1854.

Critchley M: Aphasiology and Other Aspects of Language. London, Edward Arnold, 1970.

Dax M, Dax G: Lésions de la moitié gauche de l'encéphale coïncidant avec l'oubli des signes de la pensée. Lu au Congrès méridional tenu à Montpellier an 1836 par le docteur Marc Dax. Gaz Hebd Méd Chir 1865;33:259–262.

Del Litto V: Album Stendhal. Paris, Bibliothèque de la Pléiade, NRF 1968.

Doyon A: Le dossier de la mort de Stendhal. Stendhal Club 1966;33:13–17, and 1967;36:517–521.

Felman S: La " Folie" dans l'œuvre romanesque de Stendhal. Paris, 1971.

Fields WS: Historic introduction; in Ginsberg MD, Bogousslavsky J (eds): Cerebrovascular Disease, Pathophysiology, Diagnosis, and Management. New York, Blackwell Science, 1998, pp 827–833.

Fields WS, Lemak NA: A History of Stroke. Its Recognition and Treatment. New York, Oxford University Press, 1989.

Fisher CM: Intermittent cerebral ischemia; in Wright IS, Millikan CM (eds): Cerebral Vascular Disease. New York, Grune & Stratton, 1958, pp 81–97.

Heberden W: Epilepsy, head-ache, palsy, and apoplexy, and St. Vitus dance; in Commentaries on the History and Cure of Diseases. London, Payne, 1802.

Hécaen H, Dubois J: La naissance de la neuropsychologie du langage (1825–1865). Paris, Flammarion, 1969.

Hécaen H, Lanteri-Laura G: Evolution des connaissances et des doctrines sur les localisations cérébrales. Paris, Desclée de Brouwer, 1978.

Héral O: Pierre Marie Augustin Broussonnet (1761–1807), naturaliste et médecin: un cas clinique important dans l'émergence de la doctrine française des aphasies. Rev Neurol 2009;165:F45–F52.

Johnson S: Letters, quoted in McHenry LC Jr: Garrison's History of Neurology. Springfield, Thomas, 1969.

Magherini G: La Sindrome di Stendhal. Firenze, Ponte Alle Grazie, 1989.

Paciaroni M, Bogousslavsky J: The history of stroke and cerebrovascular disease; –in Handbook of Clinical Neurology, vol. 92 (3rd series) Stroke, part 1, 2009, pp 3–28.

Pinel P: Traité médico-philosophique sur l'aliénation mentale ou la manie. Paris, Richard, Caille et Ravier, An IX [1802].

Ombredane A: L'aphasie et l'élaboration de la pensée explicite. Paris, PUF, 1951.

Schiller F: Paul Broca. London, University of California Press, 1979.

Stendhal: Correspondance, tome III (1835–1842). Paris, Bibliothèque de la Pléiade, NRF, 1968.

Stendhal: Journal (1801–1823; 1818–1842); in Œuvres intimes, tome I and II. Paris, Bibliothèque de la Pléiade, 1955–1982.

Viets HR: Aphasia as described by Linnaeus and as painted by Ribeira. Bull Hist Med 1943;13:328–333.

Von Swieten G: Of the apoplexy, palsy and epilepsy. Commentaries upon the aphorisms of Dr Herman Boerhaave. London, Knapton, 1754.

Julien Bogousslavsky, MD
Center for Brain and Nervous System Disorders, and Neurorehabilitation Services
Genolier Swiss Medical Network, Clinique Valmont
CH–1823 Glion/Montreux (Switzerland)
Tel. +41 21 962 3700, Fax +41 21 962 3838, E-Mail jbogousslavsky@valmontgenolier.ch

Bogousslavsky J, Hennerici MG, Bäzner H, Bassetti C (eds): Neurological Disorders in Famous Artists – Part 3. Front Neurol Neurosci. Basel, Karger, 2010, vol 27, pp 143–159

·······················

The Missing Hands of Blaise Cendrars

Laurent Tatu

Departments of Neuromuscular Diseases and Anatomy, CHU Jean-Minjoz, University of Franche-Comté, Besançon, France

Abstract

The life and works of Blaise Cendrars (1887–1961), one of the greatest French literary authors of the 20th century, were profoundly influenced by neurology. Having been wounded in the Great War in 1915, his right forearm was amputated, and he very quickly began to suffer from stump pain and phantom hand phenomena, which persisted until his death. Following his amputation he became a left-handed writer. Half a century later, between 1956 and his death in 1961, he suffered two strokes which gradually paralyzed the left side of his body. After the second stroke in 1958, he became a 'handless writer', also partially losing his ability to express himself orally. Although the works of Blaise Cendrars portray characters with serious mental disorders, they also contain characters with real neurological diseases, such as the trepanated aphasic in 'J'ai Saigné'. The most famous of these is undoubtedly Moravagine, the protagonist of the eponymous novel, who presents acute behavioral disturbances. We learn from the autopsy report that he was in fact suffering from a brain tumor. On several occasions, including the complex case of Moravagine, and by presenting his ideas on hysteria, Blaise Cendrars, in his own way, addressed the somewhat fuzzy boundary that exists between psychiatry and neurology.

Copyright © 2010 S. Karger AG, Basel

Blaise Cendrars, né Frédéric-Louis Sauser, was one of the greatest French literary authors of the 20th century. He was born in La Chaux-de-Fonds in Switzerland on September 1, 1887. As a young innovative poet he took part in the avant-garde artistic movement in Paris, and then enlisted in the French Foreign Legion at the beginning of the Great War. He was gravely wounded in 1915 and his right forearm had to be amputated. Following his voluntary enlistment, he became a French citizen in 1916. His experience in the Great War had a permanent impact on his work and forced him to become a left-handed writer who suffered from amputee pain and phantom hand phenomena which persisted until his death.

Fifty years later, between 1956 and his death on January 21, 1961, he suffered two strokes which gradually deprived him of the use of the left side of his body, and he then became a 'handless writer'. He also gradually lost his ability to express himself orally due to a serious case of dysarthria.

Thus neurological pathologies not only had a profound physical impact on Blaise Cendrars, but they also played an important role in his work. The trepanated aphasic in 'J'ai Saigné' and, of course, Moravagine with his brain tumor, are two of the most salient examples.

Blaise Cendrars was fascinated by nervous disorders and even began studying medicine in 1908 at Waldau Psychiatric Clinic near Bern. Through the complex case of Moravagine and by presenting his ideas on hysteria, Blaise Cendrars in his own way addressed the somewhat fuzzy boundary that exists between psychiatry and neurology.

The Appearance of a Phantom Hand

When the Great War began, the young poet Blaise Cendrars had already published his first great poem, 'Les Pâques à New York' in 1912, and his first 'livre simultané' entitled 'La Prose du Transsibérien et de la Petite Jehanne de France' in 1913. He had close ties with a number of Parisian avant-garde artists including Guillaume Apollinaire (1880–1918).

On August 2, 1914, Blaise Cendrars and the Italian writer Ricciotto Canudo (1877–1923) placed an advertisement in several newspapers calling for non-French citizens living in France to enlist in the French army to fight against Germany. Having voluntarily enlisted, Blaise Cendrars was drafted into a regiment in the French Foreign Legion which involved an initial period of military instruction in Paris. In September 1914, whilst on military leave, he married Féla Poznanska, the mother of his three children Rémy, Odilon and Miriam. At the end of November 1914, his regiment set out for the Somme battlefields where Cendrars came into contact with atypical soldiers who, like him, had enlisted voluntarily and often acted outside the regular army. In September 1915, now a corporal, Cendrars and his regiment went to fight on the Champagne battlefields. During the attack on September 28, 1915, his right arm was seriously injured and the forearm had to be amputated. Cendrars' war may have had an unusual beginning, but unfortunately it had a much more classic ending comprising an injury, a stay in a military hospital and military decorations (fig. 1).

Blaise Cendrars often recalled his memories of being a soldier in the Great War in narratives such as 'La Main Coupée' (The Severed Hand), 'L'Homme Foudroyé' (The Astonished Man), 'L'Égoutier de Londres' (The London Sewer Worker) and 'J'ai Tué' (I Have Killed), but he never wrote about his injury. Even

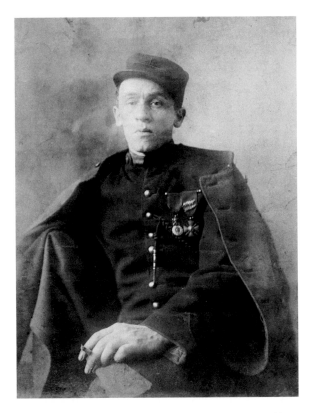

Fig. 1. Blaise Cendrars wearing his military uniform and decorations, shortly after the amputation of his right arm. Blaise Cendrars Collection, Swiss National Library, Bern. ©Miriam Cendrars.

'La Main Coupée' does not broach the subject of his injury and amputation and, according to Claude Leroy, remains 'a narrative which will never fit with its title' [Leroy, 1995, p 204]. In the first drafts of this work, Blaise Cendrars considered recounting the story of his injury and hospitalizations. But the drafts did not progress beyond the planning stage, remaining phantom descriptions of the appearance of a phantom hand [Blaise Cendrars Collection, Bern, Swiss National Library, O 170].

The only known account of the episode occurred amidst the hell of a needless offensive and was described in a letter addressed to Blaise Cendrars in 1952 by one of the soldiers in his squadron: 'The last time we saw each other was when we were both wounded and in search of the rescue station. You with your arm, wanting me to finish severing it off' [Robert Delort's letter, Blaise

Cendrars Collection, Bern, Swiss National Library, O 174]. It has been suggested that Blaise Cendrars may have cut off his right hand himself by severing it from his forearm. This theory was put forward in 1947 by his friend the writer Jacques-Henri Lévesque: 'On the battlefield, he himself [cut] off his right hand, which was still hanging from his bloodstained arm by a few shreds of flesh. You amputate just above the right elbow' [Lévesque, 1947, p 43]. The writer Florent Fels (1893–1977) proposed the same hypothesis: 'Blaise [took] a shell to the right arm, and with a trench knife [cut] off his dead and, from then on, useless hand' [Fels, 1962, p127].

The wounded Blaise Cendrars was evacuated to a surgical unit behind the lines where his right forearm was surgically amputated. In 'J'ai saigné', which was published in 1938, and is the only narrative about this period, the story begins 48 hours after the amputation. In the following extract, Cendrars is naked on a stretcher in the courtyard of a factory that has been converted into a rescue station, and awaits evacuation by ambulance to a hospital behind the lines. The stump pain is already acute and will never again leave him: '… and my severed arm was so painful that I was biting my tongue to stop myself from screaming, and now and then, long shivers shook me for I was cold in the rain, completely naked, lying on my narrow stretcher, immobile, stiff, unable to move at all, apprehensive as I was, like a mother with her newborn, about the huge bandage, which was the size of a baby, held close to my flank, this strange thing which I could not move without stirring up a universe of pain, or hold in my good hand without the big white swab becoming soaked with red, feeling an atrocious burning, and realizing that my life was escaping me, was slipping away, drop by drop, and I could do nothing to stop it because you can't stop your heart, and my heart was beating regularly, with every beat sending out a flow of blood that I could feel, as if I could see it, squirting out of my severed arm – and with these pulsations, which were morally and physically unbearable, I was able to measure time, which, alone amidst the terror of that awful night, of which I registered every detail, passed unrelentingly, its true nature consisting of seconds, fractions of seconds, eternity' [Cendrars B, 2003b, p182].

The Discarded Prosthesis

Cendrars' narratives from his period of military hospitalization, which lasted until May 1916, are rare. Military archives, however, have enabled his hospital pathway to be pieced together [French Army Military Hospital Archives, Limoges]. It began on the night of October 1st, 1915, with his admission into an auxiliary hospital in Châlons-sur-Marne, where he remained for 3 weeks. The bandages from his amputation were regularly changed. Despite the

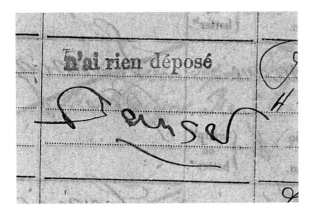

Fig. 2. The first known example of Cendrars' signature with his left hand (signing his real name 'Sauser') dating from his admission to Sceaux Military Hospital in October 1915. French Army Military Hospital Archives, Limoges.

stump pain he began his own personal rehabilitation which proved effective. He boxed into a pillow with his stump for 15 min every morning. He juggled with oranges and all sorts of other objects. Although these exertions made his stump bleed, they helped him to regain the use of his right arm. He also gradually learned to use his left hand.

On October 22, 1915, he was transferred to the Sceaux Military Hospital, on the premises of the Lakanal College in the Parisian suburbs (fig. 2). On November 2, 1915, Blaise Cendrars told his friend the poet Guillaume Apollinaire (1880–1918) about his injury: 'I was wounded on September 28th in Champagne in front of the Navarin farm during the attack on the trench of Kultur! My right arm had to be amputated. Things are going as well as possible. My mood is good' [Caizergues, 1988, p 100]. Several days later, he wrote to another friend, the Basel-born sculptor August Suter: 'You are right, two legs and one hand are enough. I have already learned to use my left hand for every-thing. From now on I will use nothing else. Through spirit and courage, I feel full of life. I still have trouble writing. Also, I won't be able to work for a while. It's a shame because I want to. Everything is fine' [Cendrars B, 1969, p 399].

At the end of 1915, he received two French military decorations, the 'Croix de guerre' and the 'Médaille militaire'. His condition improved but he still required a second operation on his upper limb in February 1916, a few days after his French naturalization was granted. Whether the reasons for this second operation were related to an infection, neuroma or scarring is unknown. It led to the definitive stump at the end of lower third of his right arm. On February

23, Cendrars wrote to August Suter: 'I have had another operation. Everything is going well now. And I am going to head down south' [Cendrars B, 1969, p 404]. On March 6, 1916, he was actually transferred for convalescence to the Maison-Blanche Hospital, a neuropsychiatric center with a special department for amputees in Neuilly-sur-Marne. He remained there until May 19, 1916, then returned home to Paris.

Blaise Cendrars experienced the use of a prosthetic right forearm. The military provided him with an initial rudimentary model. In May 1916, he wrote: 'I have a nice mechanical arm which works by itself. I am in good health, good spirits too; I am working' [Cendrars B, 1969, p 405]. However, the stump pain prevented him from wearing the prosthesis, so he abandoned it. The writer Maurice Barrès (1862–1923) provided him with a more sophisticated model, which was no more successful. Blaise Cendrars was still in pain and disagreed with even the mere idea of a mechanical limb, as explained in 1922 by one of Cendrars' great friends, the writer Albert t'Serstevens (1885–1974): 'Maurice Barrès gave him a marvelous orthopedic device, an arm made of ash wood and aluminum which, with the slightest pressure, clenched the fingers on their metallic hinges. For a while, Cendrars enjoyed using the contraption in front of his friends, but he then became disgusted by this mechanical limb. He just abandoned [it] in a station; when he was going on a trip, he deposited it at the left luggage office, thus lightening his load' [t'Serstevens, 1972, pp 414–415].

The subject of the prosthesis appears several times in the works of Blaise Cendrars. The dialogue between Chaude-Pisse, the surname of Garnero, a soldier in his squadron, and Blaise Cendrars in 'La Main Coupée' is one example: '– So then Chaude-Pisse, you don't have a wooden peg? – I've even got an American leg, but I only put in on a Sunday to go to the cinema. I left my wooden peg in the car, my stump is hurting. –That's like me, you see, my sleeve is empty. I can't wear any contraption, my stump hurts. – What a lovely gift we've been given' [Cendrars B, 2002, p 85].

Shiva's Hands

Blaise Cendrars did not write during the Great War, with the exception of three short poems called 'Schrapnells' in October 1914. In January 1916, whilst in full rehabilitation, Blaise Cendrars began writing again. He embarked upon his new career as a left-handed writer. His 'main amie' replaced his missing hand. He produced his first manuscripts with great physical difficulty. 'Notre grande offensive. Quelques villages de la Somme. Souvenirs d'un amputé' is made up of several manuscript pages written with his left hand, alternating with pages written by a third party [Cendrars B, 1969, pp 400–403] (fig. 3). In 1916,

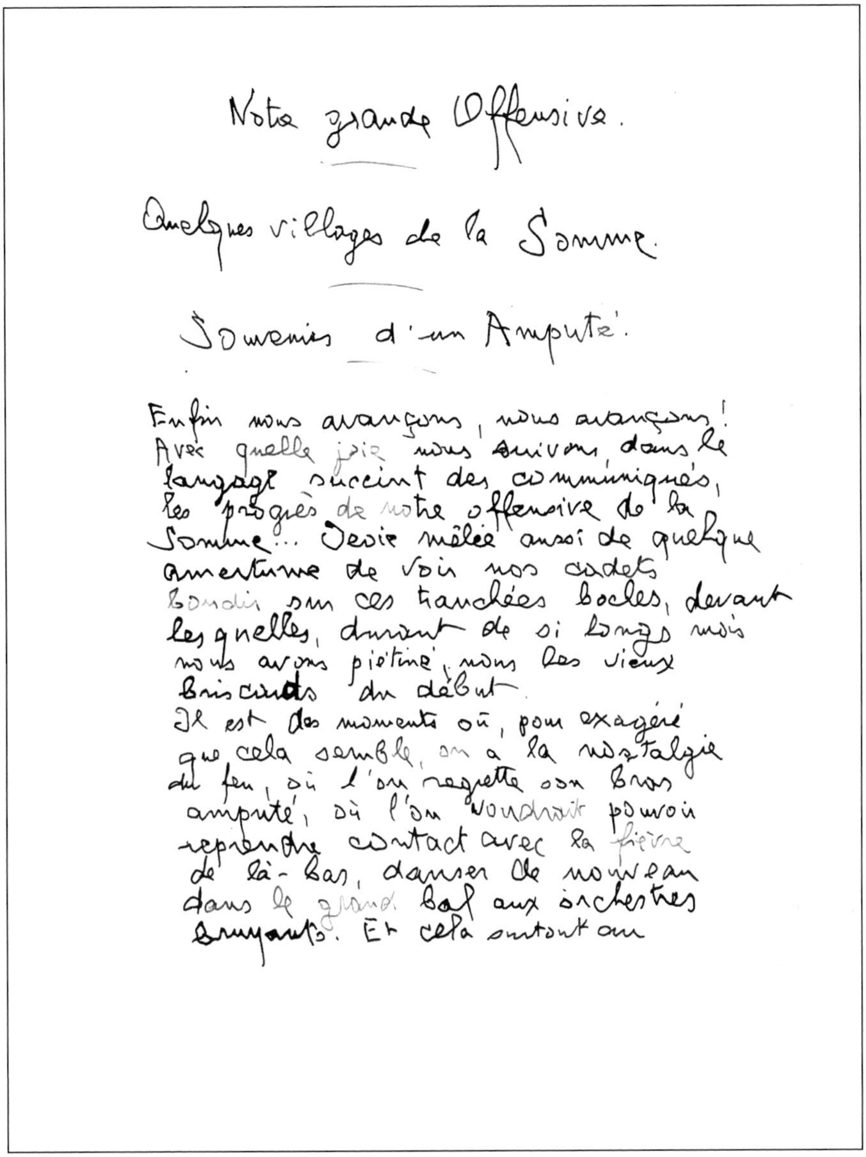

Nota grande Offensive.

Quelques villages de la Somme.

Souvenirs d'un Amputé.

Enfin nous avançons, nous avançons!
Avec quelle joie nous suivons, dans le
langage succinct des communiqués,
les progrès de notre offensive de la
Somme... Desie mêlée aussi de quelque
amertume de voir nos cadets
bondir sur ces tranchées boches, devant
lesquelles, durant de si longs mois
nous avons piétiné, nous les vieux
briscards du début.
Il est des moments où, pour exagéré
que cela semble, on a la nostalgie
du feu, où l'on regrette son bras
amputé, où l'on voudrait pouvoir
reprendre contact avec la fièvre
de là-bas, danser de nouveau
dans le grand bal aux orchestres
bruyants. Et cela surtout au

Fig. 3. An example of one of Cendrars' first literary endeavors with his left hand following his amputation. Blaise Cendrars Collection, Swiss National Library, Bern. ©Miriam Cendrars.

'La Guerre au Luxembourg' was the first poem published after his injury. In the years that followed, Blaise Cendrars launched into writing his two greatest novels of the post-war period: 'L'Or' (Gold), published in 1925 and 'Moravagine', published in 1926.

Even though he never wrote about the period involving his injury and amputation, Blaise Cendrars' work and personal narratives are littered with references to his amputee pain, which persisted until his death. On November 29, 1953, he made the following entry in his journal: 'Pain radiating from back to upper right lung and end of stump' [Blaise Cendrars Collection, Bern, Swiss National Library, Journal 1953–1958].

Like many other amputees of the Great War, Cendrars' pain related to the stump of his forearm and was accompanied by pain coming from his phantom hand. The most striking description of this phenomenon is undoubtedly the one given in 'Le lotissement du ciel' (Sky) in 1949: '… the mind strays, trying to follow, to situate, to identify, to localize the existence of a severed hand, which makes itself painfully felt; not at the end of the stump or in the radial axis or at the center of the consciousness, but as an aura, somewhere outside of the body, a hand, hands which multiply and grow and fan out, the fingers virtually crushed, the nerves ultrasensitive, leaving an imprint on the mind of the image of the dancing Shiva revolving under a circular blade, severing off each arm, one by one…' [Cendrars B, 2005, pp 66–67]. Evoking Shiva in this way also reflects the philosophical theme of the divine man approached in 'J'ai tué'.

Blaise Cendrars had more ambitious literary plans regarding the pain associated with the amputation (fig. 4). The discarded drafts of 'La Main Coupée' included plans for several chapters about the pain associated with both his stump and the surgery. On December 12, 1944, in a letter to Jacques-Henry Lévesque, he refers to the first draft of his book 'La Main Coupée'. The draft was of a highly medical nature and was abandoned very soon after: 'I have been writing a new book for about eight days now called La Main Coupée, an analysis of the physical pain that the docs have often asked me to write after what I told them about my hand. It's not pleasant, but it appears that the book might be useful to them (they think so) for they have never studied the pain (it's me who thinks that – with the exception of Prof. Leriche)' [Cendrars and Lévesque, 1991, p 286]. Prof. René Leriche (1879–1955) was a specialist in sympathetic surgery and pain-related phenomena, and Cendrars held him in high regard. Leriche frequently worked with former soldiers of the Great War on the pain associated with amputation. To this day, there is nothing to confirm that Blaise Cendrars ever consulted Prof. Leriche, but his interest in this surgeon's work has been confirmed on several occasions. For example, the Blaise Cendrars Collection contains a copy of a book by Drs Frederic Leclerc and Pierre Moreau called 'Les Moignons douleureux', published at the end of the 1930s. This book was

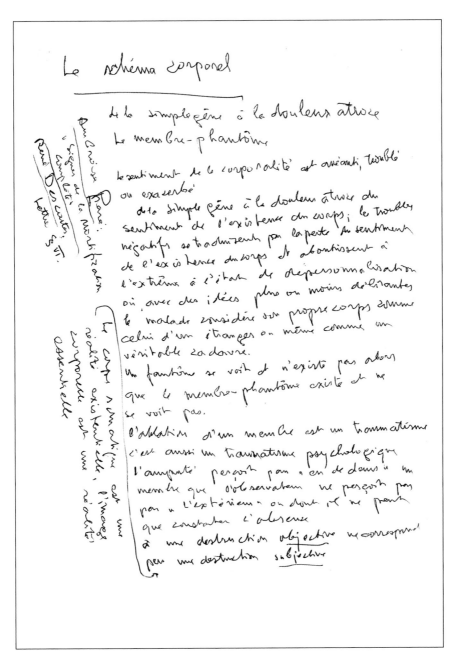

Fig. 4. Medical notes on body scheme taken by Blaise Cendrars including the following extract: 'A phantom is visible but does not exist whereas a phantom-limb exists but is invisible'. Blaise Cendrars Collection, Swiss National Library, Bern. ©Miriam Cendrars.

dedicated to Cendrars and contains a rich bibliography on the work of Leriche [Blaise Cendrars Collection, Bern, Swiss National Library, O 177].

Moravagine's Tumor

Two characters with neurological disorders in the form of cerebral lesions appear in the works of Blaise Cendrars: the trepanated soldier in 'J'ai saigné' and Moravagine. 'J'ai saigné', which recounts Cendrars' hospitalization in October 1915, describes his meeting with a wounded soldier who has undergone trepanation on two occasions. The first trepanation paralyzed his right side and the second left him aphasic. Cendrars invests greatly in helping the wounded soldier to recover his speech and describes his lengthy rehabilitation, whilst he himself is in the process of recuperating following the amputation of his right forearm. It is hard to read this narrative without seeing a premonitory vision of the two strokes that would paralyze Cendrars, depriving him of the ability to speak in the final years of his life, and of the long battle he would endure in an attempt to recover.

At first glance, Moravagine's serious mental disturbances are indicative of a psychiatric pathology and prompt research into the mentally ill patients on which Cendrars may have modeled his characters. The potential possibilities are numerous. Some of them were recalled from Cendrars' own memory, such as the voluntarily enlisted Max Starkman (1891–1915) who was killed in one of the 1915 offensives, and others were based on biographical facts such as Adolf Wölfli (1864–1930), a schizophrenic, and prominent figure in art brut, who was locked up in the Bern asylum where Cendrars could have met him [Flückiger, 2006]. The Swiss writer Jacques Chessex (1934–2009) proposed Charles-Augustin Favez, the mentally-ill character in his novel 'Le Vampire de Ropraz', as a literary model for Moravagine by imagining a fictitious meeting between Favez and Blaise Cendrars [Chessex, 2007, pp 107–110].

Despite this multiplicity of psychiatric models, it should not be forgotten that Moravagine was a character suffering from a genuine neurological disorder in the form of a nervous system lesion, or more specifically, a tumor of the third cerebral ventricle. Thus through the complex case of Moravagine, Blaise Cendrars, in his own way, addressed the somewhat blurry boundary that exists between psychiatry and neurology, and between mental disturbances and organic nervous system lesions.

The long detail given in the clinical observations on Moravagine and the results of his autopsy, which are barely comprehensible to the layperson, are the subject of the chapter entitled 'Le masque de fer' in 'Moravagine'. This very detailed medical report is virtually identical, even to the point of the footnotes, to

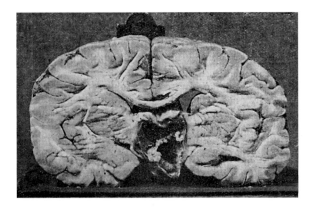

Fig. 5. Frontal brain section showing a ventricular tumor taken from Claude and Lhermitte's article. This is the patient on which Blaise Cendrars based Moravagine's autopsy report [Claude and Lhermitte, 1917].

an article published in the journal 'La Presse Médicale' on July 23, 1917, under the title 'Le syndrome infundibulaire dans un cas de tumeur du troisième ventricule' [Claude and Lhermite, 1917]. The authors of the article were the famous neurologists Henri Claude (1869–1945) and Jean Lhermitte (1877–1959), both doctors in a military neurological center at the time. Blaise Cendrars produced a very faithful reproduction of the first part of this article, but it is interesting to note the modifications that he made. One short paragraph concerning the experimental stimulation of the hypophysis was not reproduced. Cendrars changed the age and the initials of the submarine soldier in the article and turned him into an aviator. He also changed the name of the neurological center which became 'le centre 101 bis' in the novel, and added the name of the Orinoco river to the medical observations cited in the novel. More curiously, Blaise Cendrars systematically reduced the volumes of the patient's diuresis in the observations so that they did not exceed 2.5 liters/day. Finally, he modified the name of the person who carried out the pathological analysis; Mademoiselle Loyez became Mademoiselle Germaine Soyez which, in the novel, is the name of the nurse who looks after Moravagine in the '101 bis' neurological center (fig. 5).

Cendrars and Hysteria

Blaise Cendrars very much had a love-hate relationship with psychiatry. He initially began studying medicine in 1908 in Bern to learn more about it.

Fascinated by theories of the subconscious and by the causes of nervous disorders, he enrolled at the Faculty of Medicine in Bern for the summer semester of 1908 [Cendrars M, 2006, pp. 148–157]. He chose to do his work experience at the Waldau University Psychiatric Clinic near Bern, which was transposed into 'Waldensee' in 'Moravagine'. The experience only lasted one semester. Blaise Cendrars was disappointed by the teaching and by the doctors' conceptions of illness, particularly the psychiatrists. He abandoned his medical studies [Cendrars M, 1987].

Several years later, in one of the first drafts of 'Moravagine' dating from August 1, 1917, the following negative phrase appeared alongside the future chapter title 'Internat': 'issue a terrible indictment against the psychiatrists and experimentally determine their psychology' [Blaise Cendrars Collection, Bern, Swiss National Library, O 67]. In order to reach this objective, in the final version of the novel Cendrars uses the example of hysteria, a highly contentious issue amongst neurologists, psychiatrists and psychoanalysts: 'Hysteria, the Great Hysteria, was then much in fashion in medical circles. Following the preliminary work of the schools of Montpellier and la Salpetriere, which had, so to speak, done no more than define and situate the object of their studies, a number of foreign men of science, particularly the Austrian, Freud, had taken up the problem, had gone into it more amply, more profoundly, had lifted it, extracted it from its purely experimental and clinical domain to make of it a kind of pataphysics of social, religious and artistic pathology, in which it was not so much a question of coming to know the climacteric of this or that obsession born spontaneously in the farthest regions of consciousness and determining the simultaneity of the 'auto-vibrism' of sensations observed in the subject, but rather of creating, of forging an entire system of sentimental (supposedly rational) symbolism of acquired or innate slips of the subconscious, a kind of key to dreams for use by psychiatrists, as codified by Freud in his works on psychoanalysis…' [Cendrars B, 2003a, p. 12].

The issue of hysteria and simulation, an age-old controversy, made a marked reappearance during the 1st World War, when certain soldiers suffering from war neuroses were considered to be malingerers. Blaise Cendrars was definitely directly confronted by the problem of hysteria with the soldiers in his squadron. He initially tackled the problem of masculine hysteria in 'La Main coupée' using the soldier Lang as an example: 'He was a lousy soldier. When the blues got hold of him, he was more annoying than a woman at that time of the month. He'd get a migraine, would brood, was frankly unbearable and had acute neurasthenia. Another hysteric. God, these big, strapping fellows are such cowards' [Cendrars B, 2002, p. 21].

Following his amputation, Cendrars was able to continue his contact with sufferers of war neuroses between March and May 1916 during his convalescent stay at the Maison-Blanche Hospital, which was also a neuropsychiatric center. It may have been during his stay there that Cendrars searched for inspiration for the '101 bis' neurological center in 'Moravagine' and the soldier Souriceau, who became mentally ill during the Great War.

The Paralyzed 'Main Amie'

At the end of the trying 2nd World War period, Blaise Cendrars began writing his memoires which led to the publication of four volumes: 'L'Homme Foudroyé' (1945), 'La Main Coupée' (1946), 'Bourlinguer (Planus)' (1948) and 'Le Lotissement du Ciel' (1949). In 1952, at the age of 65, Blaise Cendrars was still in good health. His body managed to cope with the generous quantities of white wine that he consumed and the two packets of cigarettes that he smoked per day [Cendrars and Miller, 1995, p. 54]. However, he had some ophthalmological problems which in 1954 required him to consult and be treated by Dr. Lucien Maussion, an ophthalmic specialist.

Time combined with the over-use of his upper left limb brought on pain of such intensity that it sometimes prevented him from being able to write. On several occasions in his correspondence he wrote of painful phenomena in the upper left limb which he sometimes qualified as 'neuritis': 'Unfortunately, I am suffering from neuritis which is almost preventing me from holding my pen' [Cendrars and Lévesque, 1991, p. 561]. In May 1956, a few months before the onset of his first stroke, he complained again of painful phenomena in his left arm, adding to his amputee pain: '…nothing can be maintained, nothing lasts, except for the age-old pain in my severed arm and the new pain in my intact left arm, which is astoundingly intense and unfamiliar. Enough is enough…' [Blaise Cendrars Collection, Bern, Swiss National Library, Journal 1953–1958].

In June and July 1956, Blaise Cendrars made several entries in his journal about the pain and heaviness that he felt in his lower limbs. He lost 5 kg in one year. On the night of July 21, 1956, at the Ouchy Château-Hôtel in Lausanne where he was on holiday, Blaise Cendrars suffered his first stroke which led to a motor deficit in the left side of his body (fig. 6). It is of course not possible to ascertain whether the stroke was ischemic or hemorrhagic in nature. One month later, he sent word to the American writer Henry Miller (1891–1980), with whom he maintained regular correspondence by dictating letters to a third party which he signed by hand: 'For one month, my left leg and arm have been paralyzed and the hand which used to command the type-writer no long obeys me. This is the worst thing that could have happened to me! A good deal of patience and goodwill will be required to overcome all of this, let's give it a year' [Cendrars and Miller, 1995, p. 285].

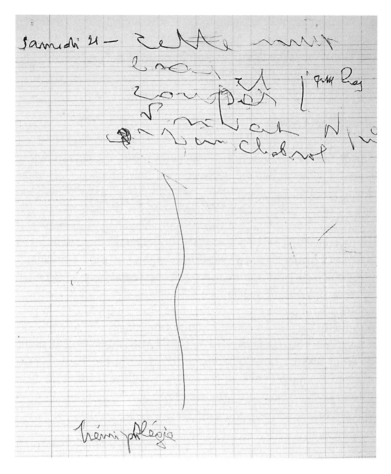

Fig. 6. Text written by Blaise Cendrars in his journal using his paralyzed left hand several hours after the onset of his first stroke on July 21, 1956. At the bottom, Cendrars manages to write the word 'hemiplegia'. Blaise Cendrars Collection, Swiss National Library, Bern. ©Miriam Cendrars.

Blaise Cendrars maintained his courage, after all he had already experienced a long rehabilitation process following the amputation of his right forearm. He knew that his body could overcome this new challenge. A kinesitherapist came several times a week and Raymone Duchâteau, who he married in 1919 after 32 years of friendship, took an active part in helping him. Prof. André Lemaire went to see him on three occasions in August 1956.

Witnesses from this period confirmed that Blaise Cendrars' will remained intact. His friend Nino Franck (1904–1988) with whom he collaborated on a series of radiophone broadcasts at the beginning of the 1950s, left the following account describing his vivacity and his desire to recuperate after his first stroke: 'After the hemiplegia, Blaise hadn't really changed. He limped a little, with a grimace at the corner of his mouth. He was as robust as a tree trunk that remains intact, even after lightning strikes. He was apparently unchanged, with from then on, the extraordinary and sweet Raymone constantly at his side to hold him up after the first drink. His speech was hardly affected. And he had regained the energy described by those who saw him after his mutilation during the war, often witnessing him exercising the joints in his left hand; the only one he had left: no more afflicted in 1958 than in 1917, he was starting again' [Franck, 1962, p 153].

Blaise Cendrars' efforts enabled him to regain sufficient strength in his upper left limb to start writing again. On September 1, 1956, the day of his 69th birthday, he made the following journal entry: 'Bit by bit, I am getting back to work. I hope to be able to hold my pen. My fourth finger is starting to move'. But the challenge continued to test him and on October 30, he still had not managed to recommence his work as a writer: 'Tomorrow, I am going to try to start writing again. Some new ones to start with!' [Blaise Cendrars Collection, Bern, Swiss National Library, Journal 1953–1958].

The Final Stroke

The process of rehabilitation after his stroke in the summer of 1956 was long and arduous. One year later, he was still unable to walk. On August 13, 1957, in a letter to Henry Miller, he wrote: 'I am better than I was a year ago, but I can't walk anymore' [Cendrars and Miller, 1995, p 287]. Over the months, Blaise Cendrars managed to go outdoors again and was able to write using his left hand in a larger, but legible, handwriting. He did not write anything new, instead deciding to work on a group of old texts called 'Trop c'est Trop'.

In the summer of 1958, Blaise Cendrars fell victim to a second stroke. The left side of his body was paralyzed again and this time, his speech was affected. The account given by Nino Franck describes a severe case of dysarthria: 'Clearly weakened, hardly speaking (the words were still there and still governed by a spirit of precision, but were so distorted that he quickly put a stop to them)' [Franck, 1962, p 153]. Cendrars obstinately continued to write but the pages of writing in his notebooks are illegible. At the end of 1958, minister and writer André Malraux (1901–1976) went to Cendrars' home to

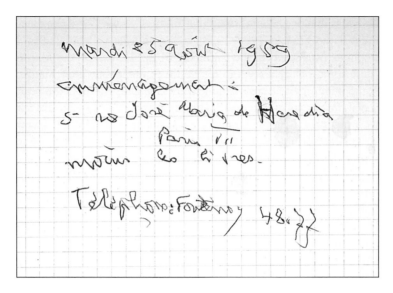

Fig. 7. One of Cendrars' final journal entries mentioning his last move to ground-floor accommodation in August 1959. Blaise Cendrars Collection, Swiss National Library, Bern. ©Miriam Cendrars.

present him with the 'cravate de commandeur' from the Legion of Honour. Blaise Cendrars found the strength to stand up for a few minutes during the ceremony.

At the beginning of 1959, Blaise Cendrars asked Nino Franck to help him type up one of his texts: 'I sat down in front of his old type-writer. Blaise was holding a notebook in his hand. I suggested to him that, to avoid tiring himself out by dictating, he leave me to decipher what he had written. He refused: it was illegible to anyone but him' [Franck, 1962, p 154]. This text, which is several pages in length, is about his memories of a trip to Rome, and was Cendrars' final narrative [Cendrars M, 2006, pp 683–688].

Blaise Cendrars and Raymone moved for the last time into a ground floor apartment to enable Blaise to benefit from going outside from time to time (fig. 7). Albert t'Serstevens was amongst those who visited Cendrars in the final months. He found a shriveled, petrified, silent man, with skeletal features. Dr. Jean Chabrol, the husband of one of Raymone's cousins and Blaise's general practitioner, also came to see him regularly. Blaise Cendrars' health deteriorated over the winter of 1960. He died on January 21, 1961, after having received in extremis his only official literary award whilst living, namely the 'Grand Prix Littéraire de la ville de Paris'.

Acknowledgements

I would like to give particular thanks to: Miriam Cendrars for her invaluable help and providing information on her father's medical history; Marie-Thérèse Lathion curator of the Blaise Cendrars Collection at the Swiss National Library (Bern) for her time and availability, and her help with the illustrations; Jean-Carlo Flückiger, Director of the Centre d'Études Blaise Cendrars (CEBC) at the Swiss National Library (Bern) for his helpful advice; Julien Bogousslavsky for once again sharing his vast literary knowledge with me, and Melanie Cole for revising the English text.

References

Caizergues P: Blaise Cendrars et Apollinaire; in Actes du colloque "Modernités de Blaise Cendrars". Revue littéraire Sud, 1988, pp 71–102.
Cendrars B: Inédits secrets. Paris, Le Club français du livre, 1969.
Cendrars B: La Main coupée. Tout autour d'aujourd'hui – Œuvres complètes tome 6. Paris, Denoël, 2002.
Cendrars B: Moravagine. Tout autour d'aujourd'hui – Œuvres complètes tome 7. Paris, Denoël, 2003a.
Cendrars B: J'ai saigné; in Histoires vraies. Tout autour d'aujourd'hui – Œuvres complètes tome 8. Paris, Denoël, 2003b.
Cendrars B: Le Lotissement du ciel. Tout autour d'aujourd'hui – Œuvres complètes tome 12. Paris, Denoël, 2005.
Cendrars B, Lévesque JH: J'écris. Écrivez-moi. Correspondance (1924–1959). Paris, Denoël, 1991.
Cendrars B, Miller H: Correspondance 1934–1979: 45 ans d'amitié. Paris, Denoël, 1995.
Cendrars M: Blaise Cendrars. La Vie, le Verbe, l'Écriture. Paris, Denoël, 2006.
Cendrars M: Waldensee ou Waldau; in Le Premier siècle de Cendrars 1887–1987. Paris, Cahiers de sémiotique textuelle, 1987, pp 103–108.
Chessex J: Le Vampire de Ropraz. Paris, Grasset, 2007.
Claude H, Lhermitte J: Le syndrome infundibulaire dans un cas de tumeur du troisième ventricule. La Presse médicale, 23 juillet 1917, pp 417–418.
Fels F: Le lansquenet Cendrars; in Mercure de France mai 1962, pp 123–130.
Flückiger J-C: Histoires d'un livre; in Blaise Cendrars sous le signe de Moravagine. Caen, Lettres modernes Minard, 2006, pp 15–41.
Franck N: Une mort difficile; in Mercure de France, mai 1962, pp 144–157.
Leroy C: La Main de Cendrars. Villeneuve d'Ascq, Presses universitaires du Septentrion, 1996.
Lévesque J-H: Blaise Cendrars. Paris, Éditions de la nouvelle revue critique, 1947.
t'Serstevens A: L'Homme que fut Blaise Cendrars. Paris, Denoël, 1972.

Prof. Laurent Tatu, MD
Departments of Neuromuscular Diseases and Anatomy, CHU Jean-Minjoz
University of Franche-Comté, Boulevard Fleming
FR–25030 Besançon (France)
Tel. +33 3 81 66 82 48, Fax +33 3 81 66 80 21, E-Mail laurent.tatu@univ-fcomte.fr

Bogousslavsky J, Hennerici MG, Bäzner H, Bassetti C (eds): Neurological Disorders in Famous Artists – Part 3. Front Neurol Neurosci. Basel, Karger, 2010, vol 27, pp 160–167

. . . .

Visual Experiences of Blaise Pascal

Maurizio Paciaroni

Stroke Unit and Division of Cardiovascular Medicine, University of Perugia, Perugia, Italy

Abstract

The writings of Blaise Pascal (1623–1662), mathematician, physicist, and theologian, are often thought of as an ideal example of classical French prose. In fact, Pascal's scientific contributions include the principle of hydrostatics, known as Pascal's Law. In mathematics, he helped develop the probability theory and also made significant contributions to the realization of infinite series and the geometry of curves. He is also considered one of the most important French philosophers principally due to his book entitled 'Pensées'. Pascal had a religious conversion in the 1650s and following this he devoted himself more to religion than science. There is evidence that Pascal suffered from visual migraines with recurring headaches, episodes of blindness in half of his visual field, zigzag, fortification spectra, and other visual hallucinations. It is believed that the migraine aura experiences might have acted as a source of inspiration for Pascal's philosophical reflections. Pascal's sudden religious conversion, probably the most decisive moment in Pascal's personal life, during the night of the 23rd to 24th of November 1654, was accompanied by a lighted vision which he interpreted as fire which brought him the total conviction of God's 'reality and presence'. This experience may have been based on the effects of a migraine aura attack. In fact, this spiritual experience led him to dedicate the rest of his life to religious and philosophical interests.

Copyright © 2010 S. Karger AG, Basel

René Onfray wrote about Pascal: 'Perhaps he had a scintillating scotoma followed by a migraine that memorable night of November 23 when he wrote the parchment found after his death sewn in his garment. In the center he wrote "fire" and he made a note of the time of the crisis, from about 10.30 p.m. to 12.30 a.m.: the lines are unfinished and certain words illegible. Surely Pascal had that evening an entirely spiritual illumination, but it is not inconceivable that this sudden religious clarity, which moved him to tears, appeared to him during his migrainous insomnia' [Onfray, 1926; Podoll and Robinson, 2002]. This 'fire' experience was a source of inspiration for Pascal's philosophical and religious reflections.

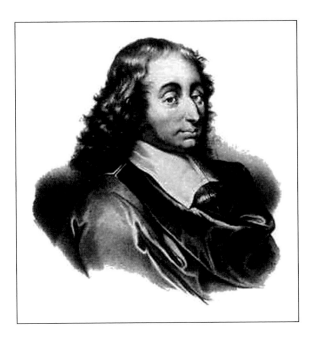

Fig. 1. Blaise Pascal.

Brief Life of Blaise Pascal (1623–1662)

Blaise Pascal (fig. 1), the French religious philosopher, mathematician, physicist, and master of prose, is considered one of the great minds of the Western intellectual world. Pascal was born in Clermont-Ferrand on June 19, 1623, and was the third of Étienne Pascal's children and his only son. Blaise's mother died when he was only 3 years old and in 1631 the family moved to Paris. Blaise Pascal's father, a local judge at Clermont, had unorthodox educational views and decided to teach his son himself. Blaise soon proved himself a mathematical prodigy but his father decided that Blaise was not to study mathematics before the age of 15 and all mathematics texts were removed from their house. Blaise however, insatiably curious about mathematics, started to work on geometry himself at the age of 12 discovering that the sum of the angles of a triangle are two right angles. At the age of 16, he formulated one of the basic theorems of projective geometry, known as Pascal's Theorem and described it in his 'Essay on Conic Sections' published in February 1640 (Essai pour les coniques) [Pascal, 1939] that Descartes refused to believe had been written by one so young. In the same year, the family moved to Rouen. Two years later, Pascal began working on his calculating machine. In fact, he invented the first digital calculator to help his father with his work which involved collecting taxes. Blaise worked on this invention for 3 full years between 1642 and 1645. This device, called the 'Pascaline', resembled a mechanical calculator later found in the 1940s. This, almost certainly, makes Pascal the second person to invent a mechanical calculator for Schickard had manufactured one in 1624 [O'Connor and Robertson, 1996]. In conjunction with the French mathematician Pierre de Fermat, Pascal was also responsible for formulating the mathematical theory of probability, which has become important in such fields as actuarial, mathematical, and social statistics, not to mention a fundamental element in the calculations of modern theoretical physics. Pascal's other important scientific contributions include the derivation of Pascal's Law or Principle, which states that fluids transmit pressures equally in all directions, and his investigations in the geometry of the infinitesimal. He also demonstrated how the weight of the earth's atmosphere balanced the mercury in the barometer by repeating Torricelli's experiments. Pascal's methodology reflected his emphasis on empirical experimentation as opposed to analytical, a priori methods. He also believed that human progress is perpetuated by the accumulation of scientific discoveries resulting from such experimentation.

Pascal was a contemporary and rival of René Descartes, the most prominent mathematician-philosopher of his day. In 1646, Pascal began a series of experiments on atmospheric pressure. By 1647 he had proved to his satisfaction that vacuum existed. Descartes visited Pascal on September 23. Pascal seemed to think that Descartes could help him with his medical problems but during this 2-day visit, the two argued about the vacuum which Descartes did not believe in. Descartes wrote, rather cruelly, in a letter to Huygens after this visit that Pascal 'has too much vacuum in his head'. The following morning, however, he returned – not Descartes the philosopher, but Descartes the physician. He sat and listened for 3 hours at his patient's side, listening to his complaints, examined him, prescribed soup and rest. When Pascal was tired of staying in bed, Descartes claimed, he would be nearly well. Their views remained in disagreement but it was the supreme rationalist in his role as thoughtful doctor whom Pascal would later remember. Later, Pascal wrote: 'The heart has its reasons which reason knows nothing of' [Sorel and Sorel, 1996].

The beginning of Pascal's spiritual transformation initiated in 1646. Pascal was raised as a Roman Catholic and had a vibrant faith in Jesus Christ, and he later became an influential Christian philosopher. He contested Descartes' view that human reason reigns supreme, arguing that it is not capable of dealing with metaphysical problems. In fact, Pascal was influenced by the teachings of the Jansenists, a heretical Catholic movement which stressed God's grace in salvation and the importance of leading a lifestyle consistent with one's faith

[Morris, 1992]. In the summer of 1647, he moved back to Paris. In 1650, he suddenly abandoned his favorite pursuits to study religion [Rouse Ball, 1908]. Sometime around then, he nearly lost his life in an accident. The horses pulling his carriage bolted and the carriage was left hanging over a bridge above the river Seine. Although he was rescued without any physical injury, it does appear that he suffered great psychological trauma. Always having been somewhat of a mystic, he considered this a special summons to abandon the world. He wrote an account of the accident on a small piece of parchment which for the rest of his life he carried on his heart to perpetually remind him of his covenant. After this mystical experience, he had another religious conversion on November 23–24, 1654, in which he fully committed himself to God. Evidence of this can be found in his writings which from that date on were of a predominantly philosophical nature. In 1656, Pascal finished the 'Provinciales', a series of letters on religion (fig. 2). Towards the end of his life, Pascal began to write and gather notes for a book on Christian apologetics. Unfortunately, because of an undiagnosed illness Pascal died on August 19, 1662, before he was able to complete the project. His passing had been thought to be the result of a terribly painful malignant stomach ulcer but Pascal's autopsy revealed a severe brain lesion (probably carcinomatous meningitis). Despite the autopsy, the cause of his continuous poor health was never precisely determined, though speculation focused on tuberculosis, stomach cancer, or a combination of the two. A few years after his death his notes, a collection of personal thoughts on human suffering and faith in God, were published. The book was entitled 'Pensées sur la religion' which means 'Thoughts on religion', and it was considered the first example of the best French literature [Pascal, 1966]. This work was published 8 years after his death by the Port Royal community in a thoroughly garbled and incoherent form. A reasonably authentic version first appeared in 1844 and it is widely considered to be a masterpiece and a landmark in French prose.

Interpretation of Visual Migraine Aura Symptoms as Divine Revelation

Remarkably, Pascal was able to achieve his extraordinary body of work despite having been in poor health since childhood. Constitutionally delicate, from the age of 17 or 18 he suffered from insomnia and acute dyspepsia. Furthermore, he suffered recurring severe headaches from his 20s onward and was troubled by a number of unusual nervous ailments in later life that left him hardly a day without pain, leading some of his contemporaries to speculate that he was in fact insane. In 1647, a paralytic attack disabled him so severely that he could not walk without crutches. His head ached, his bowels burned, his legs and feet were continually cold and wearisome aids were required to help circulate

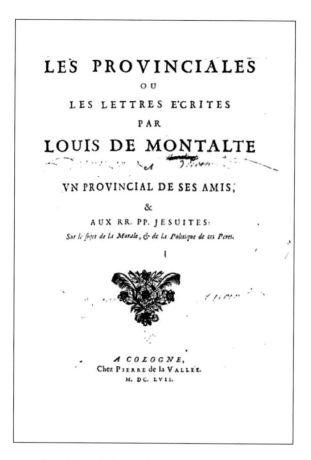

Fig. 2. Frontispiece of 'Les Provinciales', a series of letters on religion. Cologne, Pierre de la Vallée, 1657.

his blood; specifically, he wore stockings steeped in brandy to warm his feet. In part, due to this medical treatment, his health improved but his nervous system was permanently damaged. As result, he became irritable, subject to fits of proud and imperious anger and seldom smiled. In a report published in 1899 by Benoit, the Pascal's disease was described: 'Pascal suffered from neurasthenia, in that he complained frequently of transitory paraplegia, general prostration, persistent digestive disturbances and obstinate headache. He was extremely emotional, at times hypochondriacal and had many phobias with hallucinations' [Benoit, 1899]. It was not until Onfray's study [1926] which held that Pascal's visual migraines were responsible for some of his more bizarre experiences that suspect of his insanity were dismissed [Podoll and Robinson, 2002]. For some experts, the headaches which afflicted Pascal are generally attributed to his brain lesions. In this context, it is relevant to note that Pascal's sudden religious conversion, the most decisive moment in Pascal's life, during the night of November 23–24, 1654, was accompanied by light vision which he interpreted as fire. This led to his total conviction of God's reality and presence. Pascal believed this to be the beginning of a new life. In his memorial he wrote: 'Fire/God of Abraham, God of Isaac, God of Jacob/not of the philosophers and the scientists./Certainty. Certainty' [Fischer, 1971]. This experience may have been due to the effects of migraine and given spiritual significance by him, similar to the religious visions of Hildegard of Bingen [Podoll et al., 2009]. The Critchley [1967] records also reported on Blaise Pascal's strange illusions, explaining that they may have been manifestations of migraine. These unusual illusions consisted of a sudden apprehension of a cavity or yawning precipice on his left side. Also, Pascal produced manuscripts with an extraordinary broad right margin, and in places he would insert peculiar zigzag designs reminiscent of migrainous teichopsiae. These episodes may have been of a homonymous hemianopic nature, not uncommon in migraine. But despite their euphonious attribution by his contemporaries as 'l'Abîme de Pascal', it is uncertain whether or not they were of migrainous nature [Pearce, 1986]. Looking at the original manuscript of Pascal's 'Thoughts on Religion', a facsimile of which was edited by Léon Brunschvicg [1939], confirms Onfray's [1926] observation of wide right margins, which indicates blindness in half of his visual field as he was writing these pages. His handwriting on these pages is poor and sometimes illegible when compared with other samples of his writing. This impaired ability to write highly suggests symptoms of migraine with aura. The drawing in Folio 20 of the original manuscript from 'Thoughts on Religion' was considered by Onfray to represent 'an absolute proof' of Pascal's visual migraine aura experiences. He wrote: 'On page 20 of the manuscript, on a sheet of paper where not a single word is written down, there is a drawing composed of two parts, at the upper right zigzags like those which migraineurs see, and a little deeper down, in the center, a constellation of signs and bars which recall both the letters that are dancing and the luminous spots that are fluttering about in the visual field obscured at the beginning of the attack'. Onfray's interpretation is that zigzags in the upper right corner of the picture and also the pattern of predominantly curved forms in the lower half represent a visual migraine aura experience [Podoll and Robinson, 2002]. The pattern in the lower half of Pascal's drawing is similar to a migraine aura drawn by Ahlenstiel and Kaufmann [1953] that shows multiple rows of basic shapes. Regular patterns like those in Pascal's drawing, although much rarer than the common zigzags of fortification spectra, can nevertheless be experienced as visual hallucinations during a migraine [Podoll and Robinson, 2002].

Migraine Aura Experience: A Source of Inspiration for Pascal's Philosophical and Religious Reflections

Pascal examined the problems of human existence from both psychological and theological points of view and he was among the first noteworthy philosophers to seriously question the existence of God. Perhaps the migraine aura experience might have acted as a source of inspiration for Pascal's philosophical reflections. Onfray [1926] thought this to be true for other statements that Pascal wrote: 'Suffering is the natural condition of Christians', and 'I have my fog and my fine weather within me'. Pascal was certainly aware of the potential benefits of his illness, a topic which he discussed in his 'Prière pour demander à Dieu le bon usage des maladies' (Prayer to Ask God for the Good Use of Disease) in about 1659 as he continued to suffer acute ill health. Furthermore, as a result of his forays into the realm of spirituality and after the religious conversion that was attributed to a migraine attack with aura, Pascal wrote many religious works influenced by this spiritual experience that led him to dedicate the rest of his life to religious and philosophical interests and activities. For example, in the 'Pensées sur la religion' Pascal attempted to explain and justify the difficulties of human life by the doctrine of original sin, and he contended that revelation can be comprehended only by faith, which in turn is justified by revelation. He is famous for the philosophical theorem known as the Pascal 'wager'. The Pascal 'wager' claims to prove that belief in God is rational with the following argument: 'If God does not exist, one will lose nothing by believing in him, while if he does exist, one will lose everything by not believing'. When he imagined himself arguing with somebody who was constitutionally unable to believe, Pascal could find no arguments to convince him. He concluded that belief in God could only be a matter of personal choice. This basically revolutionary approach to the problem of God's existence – it became a matter of betting – has never been officially accepted by any church.

References

Ahlenstiel H, Kaufmann R: Geometrisches Gestalten in optischen Halluzinationen. Arch Psychiat Z Ges Neurol 1953;190:503–529.

Benoit. La maladie de Blaise Pascal. J Nerv Ment Dis 1899;26:648.

Brunschvicg L: Blaise Pascal; in Charléty S (ed): Les Grandes Figures. Paris, Librairie Larousse, 1939.

Critchley M: Migraine from Cappadocia to Queen Square. First Sandoz Memorial Lecture; in Smith R (ed): Background to Migraine. London, Heinemann, 1967, pp 28–29.

Fischer R: A cartography of the ecstatic and meditative states. Science 1971;174:897–904.

Morris TV: Making Sense of It All. Grand Rapids, William B. Eerdmans, 1992.

O'Connor JJ, Robertson EF: Schickard biography; in The MacTutor History of Mathematics Archive, JOC/EFR, 1996.

Onfray R: Où l'on voit que Pascal avait des migraines ophtalmiques. Presse Mèd 1926;34:715–716.

Pascal B: Essai pour les coniques. Paris, 1939.

Pascal B: 'Pensees'. Translation by Krailsheimer AJ. London, Penguin Books, 1966.

Pearce JMS: Historical aspects of migraine. J Neurol Neurosurg Psychiatry 1986;49:1097–1103.

Podoll K, Robinson D: The migrainous nature of the vision of Hildegard of Bingen. Neurol Psychiatry Brain Res 2002;10:95–100.

Podoll K, Robinson D, Sacks O: Migraine Art. Berkeley, North Atlantic Books, 2009.

Rouse Ball WW: A Short Account of the History of Mathematics, ed 4. Dover Science, 1908.

Sorel E, Sorel NC: When Blaise Pascal met René Descartes. The Independent (London), June 15, 1996.

Dr. Maurizio Paciaroni
Stroke Unit and Division of Cardiovascular Medicine, University of Perugia
Santa Maria della Misericordia Hospital
IT–06126 Perugia (Italy)
Tel./Fax +39 75 5782765, E-Mail mpaciaroni@med.unipg.it

Bogousslavsky J, Hennerici MG, Bäzner H, Bassetti C (eds): Neurological Disorders in Famous
Artists – Part 3. Front Neurol Neurosci. Basel, Karger, 2010, vol 27, pp 168–173

Autism and Art

Ioan James

Mathematical Institute, Oxford, UK

Abstract
   The link between mild forms of autism and artistic creativity is suggested by a number
of individual cases. Here those of a well-known composer, Béla Bártok, and a famous visual
artist, Andy Warhol, are considered.

   Some degree of eccentricity used to be regarded as just part of the artistic
personality. Nowadays the possibility that this was due to some kind of personality disorder is usually considered. Psychologists are quoted on the subject, often suggesting some mild form of high-functioning autism, such as
Asperger's syndrome. Starting at the other end, when highly gifted people with
a mild form of autism show artistic ability the works of art they produce have a
distinctive character, reflecting what Happé and Frith [2009] have called 'The
Beautiful Otherness of the Autistic Mind'. Numerous famous artists of the past
have been considered by Fitzgerald [2005], James [2006] and others. Attempts
at historical diagnosis often result in controversy when experts differ and ama-
teurs also get involved. The right kind of evidence is often lacking but for the
two examples discussed here, one a musician, the other a visual artist, the evidence is quite strong. The link between the affective disorders and artistic creativity is well established [Jamison, 1993]. So is the link between mild forms of
autism and scientific, especially mathematical, creativity [Baron-Cohen, 2007].
Fitzgerald [2005] believes there is a link between mild forms of autism and
artistic creativity; if so examples like these may help us to understand what the
nature of the link might be.

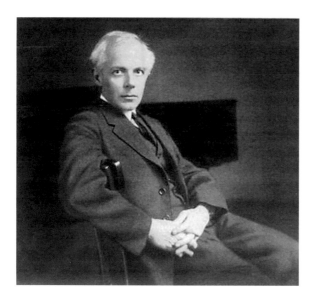

Fig. 1. Béla Bártok, 1927.

Béla Bártok

In recollections of the Hungarian musician Béla Bártok (1881–1945) we learn that his hazel eyes had a penetrating look, that his hair was white, but his face youthful in appearance (fig. 1). His normal manner was unpretentious and unassuming but at the piano he seemed like a panther in his movements, his stretchings and sudden starts. While Bártok played, it was as if all music lived in him, and the listener was impressed by his strong individuality, but when he ceased playing he returned to the remotest depths of some cavern, from which he could be drawn only by force. His piano students were sometimes driven to distraction owing to his uncompromising insistence on exactly the right turn of phrase or rhythmic realization.

Biographers have described Bártok as self-contained, introspective and showing in his writings a meticulous adherence to facts. There are references to his having been socially awkward, a man of limited conversation and possessing a probing combative nature. There is general agreement that he was a hard person to be with; few could feel really comfortable in his presence. We are told that he was 'possessed of a fanatical will and pitiless severity'; that he was 'almost painfully shy' and 'incurably nervous', that he was 'reservedly polite'. Except at the keyboard his movements often seemed to be 'hesitating and somewhat stiff', suggestive of motor clumsiness. As for peculiarities of speech and language, everyone agreed that Bártok was remarkably laconic. The intonation of his speaking voice was said to be 'exceedingly grey and monotonous'. He rarely emphasized a particular word; his words flowed out completely evenly. His voice was said to be 'excessively deep, disciplined and serene', his speech 'unusually clear, plain and at the same time, restrained, matter-of-fact and concentrated'. His letters were always written in a small clear script that looked as if every word had been put down slowly and deliberately. No time was ever wasted in courtesies, on small-talk. He knew well his own mind and self-appointed mission, and saw no virtue in circumlocution or in furthering the polite urbanities of social intercourse. As some commentators have suggested, his external brittleness functioned like a mask, which with only limited success shielded a naturally shy super-sensitive yet determined individual from the hurly-burly of the world.

When a music critic from London visited the composer at his home in Budapest he reported 'Physically as well as mentally Bártok presents striking antitheses. His loosely brushed hair is white, though his tanned face is young for his forty-four years. His strong, ruggedly rhythmical music suggests that he is big and powerful, but he is slight and lean, with hands and feet almost as delicate as a woman's. ... on the platform, at the pianoforte, he whirls tempestuously through his part; in private he is gentleness itself, alert but not aggressive, precise without being pedantic. In his grave old-world courtesy there is not a trace of affectation. One is conscious all the while of his virility, but it is of the kind that burns inwardly – that glitters through the eyes rather than expends itself in gesture, his eyes, indeed, stamp him at once as a remarkable man. They are of a rich golden brown, and he has a habit of opening them wide and slowly tilting back his head as he waits for a question'.

According to one of Bártok's professional friends, 'Whoever met Bártok, thinking of the rhythmic strength of his work, was surprised by his slight delicate figure. He has the outward appearance of a fine-nerved scholar possessed of a fanatical will and pitiless severity, and propelled by an ardent spirit, he affected inaccessibility and was reservedly polite. His being breathed light and brightness, his eyes burned with a noble fire. ... If in performance an especially hazardous and refractory passage came off well he laughed with boyish glee; and when he was pleased with the successful solution to a problem, he actually beamed'.

Although confident of the merits of his work, Bártok was not a self-publicist and began to feel he was being deprived of his due recognition. The problem was that he tended to isolate himself from people who could help him. Absorbed in his own career to the point of rudeness, he was often snubbed by those in authority and came to behave as a disgruntled internal exile. Although a dutiful and loving family man, he could not completely accommodate domestic demands that habitually had to take second place to the task at hand. In combination, this integrity and personal inflexibility caused Bártok's life to be more fraught and less immediately rewarding than it might have been.

According to Gillberg [2002] and Wolff [1995] Bártok suffered from some disorder in the autistic spectrum. Fitzgerald [2000] sees evidence of a pervasive developmental disorder. Throughout his life, he observes, Bártok focused intensely on music, although he also had a passionate interest in musical ethnology and Hungarian nationalism, believing that the future of Hungary lay in the education of the provinces. He was a workaholic who believed that a task once started always needed to be finished. He imposed great demands on his students and colleagues. It would appear that his ability to focus intensively on very narrow interests assisted his creativity. On the negative side his problems with social relationships inhibited his professional progress in the wider social world.

Andy Warhol

The American Andy Warhol (1928–1987) was enormously successful as a commercial artist in New York in the 1950s. In 1960 he began making paintings based on mass-produced images such as newspaper advertisements and comic strips. His paintings of Campbell's soup cans were such a sensational success and Warhol soon found himself the most famous and controversial figure in American Pop Art. His celebrity, carefully cultivated by himself, came as much from his lifestyle as from his work.

The composer Ian Stewart, in an unpublished lecture, made out the case for Warhol having had some form of autism. Stewart explained that what first convinced him was the chapter 'Underwear Power' Warhol wrote in 1975. 'I think underwear must be especially problematic for people who are autistic', Stewart (who has autism himself) remarked, 'because I have to get exactly the same type from the same high street shop year in year out and I'm sure green underwear feels different from other colors'. For Warhol, it was necessary to examine even the label on the packaging to make sure nothing had changed, such as the washing instructions. Stewart goes on to address the question of how autism affected Warhol's art. 'He was, of course an exceptional draughtsman, one of the skills often found in people with autism. … He is usually credited with introducing multiple versions of the same images in a grid pattern into art. … Such patterns are more likely to register and be of interest to someone who is autistic'.

At school Warhol showed a great talent for avoiding personal contact. 'He had no consideration for other people. He was socially inept at the time and showed little or no appreciation for anything'. 'He never had much to say and when he did talk it was always about his work. He was really wrapped up in his work'. The absolute flatness of his voice, his peculiar locutions, his inability to process human speech correctly are also indications. He cringed from physical contact. The obsessive playing of gramophone records, the collecting of furniture and objects such as cookie jars are also significant, likewise his obsessive archival activities, in which he documented his 'wrongness'. Biographers mention his tendency to establish routines, such as the regular morning and evening rounds of his collections. Far from attempting to conceal such characteristic patterns of behavior he started to exaggerate and exploit them; some of his followers copied what he did. Warhol describes himself as a loner: 'I wasn't close to anyone, I felt left out'. 'Every simple thing I do looks strange', he said. 'I have such a strange walk and a strange look. …. What's wrong with me?' He enumerated what he saw in the mirror: 'Nothing is missing. It's all there. The affectless gaze. The diffracted grace … the bored languor, the wasted pallor … the chic freakiness, the basically passive astonishment … the glamour rooted in despair, the self-admiring carelessness, the perfected otherness, the shadowy, voyeuristic, vaguely sinister aura … nothing is missing. I'm everything my scrapbook says I am. If you want to know all about Andy Warhol, just look at the surface of my paintings and films and me and there I am. There's nothing behind it'.

Fitzgerald [2005] has discussed Warhol's case. As a young adult he was described as a mixture of 6-year-old child and well-trained artist. He was very naïve and left himself open … there was something fragile and unprotected about him. He was very much a night creature and literally afraid to go to sleep at night. He was certainly narcissistic and fed his narcissism with his publicity and his control of other people. He was voyeuristic both in the specifically sexual sense and in the wider sense of a person who truly enjoyed vicariously the experience of others. He got enormous satisfaction from seeing people abusing drugs and alcohol and behaving in eccentric ways. Fitzgerald ends his profile of Warhol by saying that a very strong case can be made for the contention that he had Asperger's syndrome. He had major social relationship problems and showed a lack of empathy with people. He was a workaholic with narrowly focused interests. He showed motor clumsiness and spoke in a monotonous voice. His thinking style was mechanical; he was extremely controlling and immature in personality. He was also an artistic genius.

Some references to the literature on the link between autism and creativity, particularly artistic creativity, are given at the end of this note. Here it is hardly possible to go into the subject in depth, but Fitzgerald [2005] has suggested what the connection might be. After considering various cases he concludes that the autistic artist, because of his or her rather diffuse identity, and diffuse psychological boundaries, works in an effort to sort out their confused identities. The work is a focus of self-help or self-therapy; it can be an effort to sort out the perceptual puzzlement that they experience and to make sense of their autistic worlds. People with mild forms of autism often suffer from depression and artistic work can have an antidepressant effect. It is a form of self-expression for people who find other forms of expression difficult. They may have immature personalities, retaining a childlike view of the world around them, which helps their artistic work. It seems to me this theory fits Warhol's case better than Bártok's.

References

Baron-Cohen S, Wheelwright S, Burtenshaw A, Hobson E: Mathematical talent is linked to autism. Human Nature 2007;18:125–131.

Cooke AZ: Andy and Autism. Art News, 1999, 5.

Fitzgerald M: Did Bártok have HDA/ASP? Autism Europe Link 2000;29:21.

Fittzgerald M: Autism and Creativity. Hove, Brunner-Routledge, 2004.

Fitzgerald M: The Genesis of Artistic Creativity: Asperger's Syndrome and the Arts. London, Kingsley 2005.

Frith U (ed): Autism and Asperger Syndrome. Cambridge, Cambridge University Press, 1991.

Frith U: Autism: Explaining the Enigma. Oxford, Blackwell, 2003.

Happé F, Frith U: The beautiful otherness of the autistic mind. Philos Trans R Soc Lond B Biol Sci 2009;364:1346–1350.

James I: Asperger's Syndrome and High Achievement: Some Very Remarkable People. London, Kingsley, 2006.

Jamison KR: Touched with Fire. New York, Simon and Schuster, 1993.

Ledgin N: Asperger's and Self-Esteem: Insight and Hope through Role Models. Arlington, Future Horizons, 2002.Ratey and Johnson 1997

Walker A, Fitzgerald M: Unstoppable Brilliance: Irish Geniuses and Asperger's Syndrome. Dublin, Liberties Press, 2006

Warhol A: The Philosophy of Andy Warhol (from A to B and Back Again). San Diego, Harcourt Brace, 1975.

Wing L: The Autistic Spectrum. London, Constable, 2001.

Wolff S: Loners: the Life-Path of Unusual Children. London, Routledge, 1995.

Prof. I.M. James
Mathematical Institute
24–29 St Giles
Oxford OX1 3LB (UK)
Tel. +44 1865 73589, Fax +44 1865 273583, E-Mail imj@maths.ox.ac.uk

Bogousslavsky J, Hennerici MG, Bäzner H, Bassetti C (eds): Neurological Disorders in Famous Artists – Part 3. Front Neurol Neurosci. Basel, Karger, 2010, vol 27, pp 174–206

....

'A Man Can Be Destroyed but Not Defeated': Ernest Hemingway's Near-Death Experience and Declining Health

Sebastian Dieguez

Laboratory of Cognitive Neuroscience, Ecole Polytechnique Fédérale de Lausanne, Lausanne, Switzerland

Abstract

Ernest Hemingway is one of the most popular and widely acclaimed American writers of the 20th century. His works and life epitomize the image of the hyper-masculine hero, facing the cruelties of life with 'grace under pressure'. Most of his writings have a quasi-autobiographical quality, which allowed many commentators to draw comparisons between his personality and his art. Here, we examine the psychological and physical burdens that hindered Hemingway's life and contributed to his suicide. We first take a look at his early years, and review his psychopathology as an adult. A number of authors have postulated specific diagnoses to explain Hemingway's behavior: borderline personality disorder, bipolar disorder, major depression, multiple head trauma, and alcoholism. The presence of hemochromatosis, an inherited metabolic disorder, has also been suggested. We describe the circumstances of his suicide at 61 as the outcome of accumulated physical deterioration, emotional distress and cognitive decline. Special attention is paid to the war wound he suffered in 1918, which seemed to involve a peculiar altered state of consciousness sometimes called 'near-death experience'. The out-of-body experience, paradoxical analgesia and conviction that dying is 'the easiest thing' seemed to influence his future work. The constant presence of danger, death, and violence in his works, as well as the emphasis on the typical Hemingway 'code hero', can all be traced to particular psychological and neurological disorders, as well as his early brush with death.

A man can be destroyed but not defeated
Ernest Hemingway
The Old Man and the Sea (1952)

Ernest Miller Hemingway was born on July 21, 1899, in Oak Park (Illinois). He is one of the most popular American writers of the 20th century. When released in 1952, 'The Old Man and the Sea' sold 5,300,000 copies in 2 days. The novel earned him the Pulitzer Prize in 1953, and the Nobel Prize the following year. He is also celebrated for his short stories, a genre in which he excelled, his works as a journalist, a movie on the Spanish Civil War, his poetry and the prolific correspondence he left [Gurko, 1952].

Hemingway was a larger-than-life figure, not only a celebrated author, but also a real celebrity: 'His name was a synonym for an approach to life characterized by action, courage, physical prowess, stamina, violence, independence, and above all "grace under pressure" (…) He was, in short, the heroic model of an age' [Yalom and Yalom, 1971, p 485]. He was indeed 'a man living life to the hilt – deriving maximum value from experience – while achieving lasting work' [Bruccoli, 1986, p x], who filled his life and works with overtly masculine themes such as war, bravery, hunting, fishing, safari, sports, drinking, bullfights, and of course women. His constant bragging, machismo, and sense of competition became legendary[1]. A charitable view might be that: 'while aggrandizing himself, he aggrandized the practice of reading and writing' [Bruccoli, 1986, p xii]. However, we will see that psychologically inclined critics perceived his overt behavior more like a defense to ward off his inner demons. His overt behavior and immense success, indeed, stand in sharp contrast to his very sad ending, when crippled by health and mental problems he committed suicide. This act might have been surprising to the general public and his readers, but it ultimately revealed the very deep insults that kept growing throughout his life inside his body and mind.

What made him such a famous author? Hemingway brought a revolution in style and was a keen observer of the contemporary world and human nature. At odds with most of his preceding and contemporary writers, he perceived the value of economy in writing. He was perhaps the first American author to write as a journalist, opting for grade school-like grammar, simple words and short descriptions. This might seem like a self-defeating approach for a novelist, but it nevertheless left its mark. There is even a joke about 20th century American writers that says that they can all be categorized in two groups: those trying to write like Hemingway and those trying not to. Through its deliberate simplicity, use of short declarative sentences, and urge to eliminate the superfluous,

---

[1] Competition was everywhere in Hemingway's life, including the unlikely arena of literature: 'I started out very quiet and I beat Mr. Turgenev. Then I trained very hard and I beat Mr. De Maupassant. I've fought two draws with Mr. Stendhal, and I think I had an edge in the last one. But nobody's going to get me in the ring with Mr. Tolstoy unless I'm crazy or I keep getting better' [Bruccoli, 1986, p x].

Hemingway's style magnified the art of the dialogue and mastered the use of the understatement (e.g. in 'For Whom the Bell Tolls', we find this famous line: 'He was dead, and that was all'). For him, quite simply, 'the job of a writer is to tell what happened and how he feels about it' [Goldberg, 1997].

His style is encapsulated in what he called his 'iceberg theory', which he explained in 'Death in the Afternoon' (1932): 'If a writer of prose knows enough about what he is writing about he may omit things that he knows and the reader, if the writer is writing truly enough, will have a feeling of those things as strongly as though the writer had stated them. The dignity of movement of an iceberg is due to only one-eighth of it being above water' [Burhans, 1960, p 446]. The effect was to 'make people feel something more than they understood' [Young, 1975, p 39].

Hemingway knew how to tell a story and capture the imagination of millions of readers. The basic pattern of his stories is 'to expose a character to violence, to physical or psychological shock, or severe trial, and then to focus on the consequences' [Young, 1975, p 32].

It has been noted that all his male heroes are basically the same man [Gurko, 1952, p 373]. This is the 'code hero' (a term coined by Young [1966]), a character that exemplifies principles of honor, courage, and stamina in the face of adversity. There are rules for the Hemingway code hero: no self-analysis, no self-retreat, no sentimentality, no rationalizations or excuses, no apologies, no cowardice, no deceptive flourishes or fakery. The code hero is true only to himself, remains stoic in the face of adversity, and does not care about other's opinions. It is not enough for the Hemingway character to have integrity, virility and courage, he has to show and demonstrate it repeatedly, and of course under the toughest circumstances. He thus needs to pass through a number of tests in which he can display 'grace under pressure' (a phrase Hemingway seems to have coined himself [Parker, 1929]). Once the tests are passed, most of the time the hero dies [Gurko, 1952, p 374].

The writer himself seemed to have adopted this philosophy of life. His outlook was nonetheless quite pessimistic. As one critic wrote, for Hemingway 'life is one crisis after another. The naïveté which believes otherwise only produces disappointment, heartbreak, and, eventually, fruitless despair' [Gurko, 1952, p 373]. Vitality and action were his antidotes against the cruelties of life, which perhaps explains why Hemingway 'has sought out the death pattern wherever it appeared, on the battlefield, in the bullring, in the African jungle, in the individual consciousness, [as] only there could the full capacity of man's powers of survival be fully tested' [Gurko, 1952, p 375].

Of course, such a credo can quickly degenerate into ridicule and self-parody, as well as put oneself needlessly at risk and jeopardize one's valuable relationships. Indeed, the stakes Hemingway put for his heroes and himself were exceedingly high, nothing short of an attempt at immortality, as if men were mortal, but heroes immortal [Bocaz, 1971, p 53]. There were numerous obstacles to his idealized view of life and literature. One of which he was deeply aware of was celebrity: 'fame came welcomingly early, burgeoned, blossomed and finally bloated into a demanding burden' [Monteiro, 1978, p 287]. Other problems, however, were much more worrisome. This chapter first examines the psychological and physical burdens that hindered Hemingway's life and ultimately lead to his suicide. Special attention is paid to a particular event he experienced while he was a young volunteer engaged in the World War I, in which he suffered a wound that nearly killed him and, apparently, involved a peculiar altered state of consciousness sometimes called a 'near-death experience'. We then discuss the effects these pathobiographical features might have had on his works.

Psychological and Psychiatric Assessment

We do not have a medical assessment of Hemingway. Although he was formally examined during his stay at the Mayo Clinic shortly before his suicide, his doctor, Howard P. Rome, held to his promise to keep his files secret [Yalom and Yalom, 1971; Craig, 1995]. We thus have to rely primarily on the information that has been gathered by biographers, accounts by friends and relatives, as well as interviews, his vast correspondence and of course his published works (below we will return on the extent to which Hemingway's writings should be considered autobiographical or not).

Psychology
Hemingway's early years seem relevant to understand the emergence of such a complex individual (for a summary of psychological approaches to Hemingway, see table 1). At age three, baby Ernest reportedly claimed ''fraid of nothing!', which aptly introduces the basic psyche of the man to come. His father was a medical doctor who imposed a very strict education on his children, and whose mood was highly unstable. Dr. Clarence Hemingway frequently displayed angry outbursts, sometimes beating his son, interspersed with profound depressive episodes, and often needed 'rest cures' away from his family [Martin, 2006]. In 1928, deeply depressed by financial problems, burdened by diabetes and angina, he committed suicide with a collectible Civil War pistol. Hemingway's mother was also described as being inconsistent. Although we might never know exactly why the writer came to hate her so much, we know that Grace Hemingway was very controlling and dominated her more passive husband. For unclear reasons, Hemingway would eventually blame her for his

Table 1. Psychological portrait of Hemingway, derived from various sources, as outlined by Craig [1995, pp 1076–1077]

Hypothesis	Description
Neurosis emanating from parental dynamics	Father had mood disorders and was strict and violent Mother was dominant and sent mixed messages about gender identity and self-worth Confusing identification processes
Latent homosexuality	Excessive displays of masculinity (overcompensation) Scornful attitude towards homosexuals
Castration anxiety and unresolved oedipal conflict	Projective behaviors through hunting, fighting and interest for bullfight Defensive attitude towards women
Weak self-image	Public and idealized self-images were to be constantly and strenuously strived for and defended Need for power

father's suicide. Grace had an unstable mood and health, and suffered from headaches and insomnia. Most intriguingly, she went to some lengths to raise her son, and present him publicly, as a girl. Grace seemed to find some comfort in seeing Ernest as the twin of Marcelline, his sister. Both were dressed alike, but at the same time the mother encouraged her boy to display masculinity in sports, hunting and fishing. As one can imagine, much has been made of this anecdote from psychodynamic perspectives. Regardless of the alleged profound consequences for Hemingway's gender identity, he seemed to react with a combative attitude, crying out loud in his heart: 'Damn it, I'm *male*' [Young, 1975, p 44]. His youth was marked by feelings of anger and guilt, a taste for displaying courage, and an interest for violent imagery, firearms, and death. It seems plausible that the 'quest for masculinity' so emblematic of Hemingway's life and work had something to do with these early years [Martin, 2006, p 356]. His parents, it should be said, never encouraged or even accepted their son's writing [Fuchs, 1965, pp 433–434]. In fact, all they could make of it was that it was 'filth'.

Hemingway's psychological profile as an adult has been described by Hardy and Cull [1988] and summarized by Craig [1995, pp 1074–1076]. The writer emerges as a competitive and ambitious man of fierce independence, who frequently lied, exaggerated, and behaved childishly and egocentrically on many occasions. He required constant adulation and was prompt to destroy relationships when he found himself on egalitarian grounds or dominated by others. He often acted out of impulses to display his panache and could go to quite some lengths to make a point to an annoying interlocutor. The same authors have noted feelings of inadequacy and self-dissatisfaction, unstable masculine identity, tense relationships with his father (even after he committed suicide), hatred of his mother, need for extreme levels of stimulation, a deeply ingrained depression and suicidal tendencies present throughout his life. The key to understand Hemingway's behavior, it is concluded, is his need for overcompensating these flaws.

Hemingway's life and work interplay so closely that it has often been remarked that the author seemed to play one of his fictional characters in real life[2]. Yalom and Yalom [1971, p 487] argued that most of Hemingway's persona was in fact an 'image' he carefully built through the years to hide his deeper angst, and they questioned his authenticity by wondering 'whether a man firmly convinced of his identity would channel such a considerable proportion of his life energy into a search for masculine fulfillment' and highlighted his 'need to assert again and again a brute virility'.

Certainly his need for action and danger were signs of a deeper personality trait. Perhaps Hemingway was anhedonic, and needed an inordinate amount of stimulation to experience pleasure. He had difficulties in being alone and constantly sought to fill his life with excitement and travels [Yalom and Yalom, 1971, p 487; Brian, 1988], to the point of complaining after the 2nd World War 'of the emptiness and meaninglessness of his life without war'.

Hemingway's ego appeared disproportionally big, and he was extremely sensitive to any critique, bearing extraordinary grudges against everyone who dared question his talent and courage. As his idealized self-image and general expectations were clearly unrealistic, he inevitably 'fell short of his idealized goals' [Yalom and Yalom, 1971, p 490]. It has been argued that this discrepancy lead to disappointments, and ultimately to self-hatred and self-destructive tendencies.

---

[2] Critic Edmund Wilson was among the first to see clearly through Hemingway, already in the 1930s: 'And now, in proportion as the characters in his stories run out of fortitude and bravado, he passes into a phase where he is occupied with building up his public personality. He has already now become a legend (...); he is the Hemingway of the handsome photographs (...) with the ominous resemblance to Clark Gable (...). And unluckily – but for an American inevitably – the opportunity soon presents itself to exploit this personality for profit: he is soon turning out regular articles for well-paying and trashy magazines. (...) The most favorable thing one can say about it is that he made an extremely bad job of it, where a less authentic artist would probably have done somewhat better. The ordinary writer, when he projects himself, usually produces something which, though unlikely, is sympathetic; but Hemingway has created a Hemingway who is not only incredible but obnoxious. He is certainly his own worst-invented character' [Wilson, 1939].

Not surprisingly, a number of authors have written about Hemingway's alleged Oedipal issues, and speculated about repressed factors such as the 'death instinct', a fear of castration and impotence, guilt over his father's suicide, and even latent homosexuality [Drinnon, 1965; Young, 1966; Yalom and Yalom, 1971; Brenner, 1983; Meyers, 1984][3]. Prominent features dealt with from these perspectives were his treatment of women, father–son relationships, brotherly comradeship, as well as symbolic interpretations of his passion for bullfighting and hunting, and of course his war wound (see below), which very closely spared his genitalia, and might have lead to repeated inclusions of amputation and physical damage in his works[4]. More generally, Hemingway seemed to have been a fierce individualist and feared or repudiated everything that threatened to empower or surpass him (most notably women, psychiatrists, other authors and literary critics), and thereby revealed his deeper sense of insecurity. His father might have been a prime example for him, having committed suicide after a lifetime of being controlled by his wife. A fear of being rejected and abandoned might also have developed after the failure of his first love story on the Italian front with nurse Agnes von Kurowsky, which was a terrible blow to his self-esteem.

Most of Hemingway's behaviors have been interpreted in the light of defense mechanisms (i.e. denial, projection and sublimation) against an underlying depression and hypothesized fear of castration and feelings of guilt. He confronted reality by denying danger and self-limitations, and was hostile to individuals who displayed his own most inward weaknesses and feminine parts (all 'cowards', i.e. anyone who did not live to his idealized expectations, especially his father because he committed suicide). Drinking, hunting, fishing, sports and fighting have been seen as means to channel his aggressiveness and violence, allowing him to externalize his self-destructive thoughts. Quite perceptively, he famously said to Ava Gardner in 1954: 'Even though I am not a believer in the Analysis, I spend a hell of a lot of time killing animals and fish so I won't kill myself' [Hotchner, 1966, p 139]. These attempts at 'self-medica-

---

[3] Hemingway had his own ideas about psychoanalysts, which he described as 'those inner-searching Viennese eyes peering out from under the shaggy brows of old Dr. Hemingstein, that masterful deducer' [Meyers, 1987, p 545]. His distrust of psychological, and especially psychoanalytical, approaches loomed large. For instance, he dismissed Philip Young's influential work as 'the trauma theory of literature' [Young, 1975, p 44].

[4] This 'obsession' with amputation [Hovey, 1965, pp 462–464] might of course have originated in his war experience and the numerous dead and maimed soldiers he witnessed, but also in the fact that Hemingway's father, in his later years, was undermined by diabetes and feared the loss of a leg. Incidentally, when his brother Leicester shot himself in 1982; he was also suffering from depression and diabetes and likewise feared the amputation of one leg.

tion', however, amounted only to 'frenetic attempts to perpetuate the image he created, interlocked to form only a partially effective dam against an inexorable tide of anguish' [Yalom and Yalom, 1971, p 493].

Psychiatry

Hemingway suffered from numerous and well-documented mood swings. Biographer Carlos Baker [1969] was the first to use the diagnosis 'manic-depressive', now called bipolar disorder [see also Martin 2006, p 352; Beegel, 1998, p 380; Brian, 1988; Hardy and Cull, 1988; Jamison, 1996, pp 228–230; for disagreement see Meyers, 1987, p 544]. Manic episodes consisted in excessive energy and exhilaration, as well as grandiosity. Part of it, of course, may not necessarily be pathological but merely Hemingway playing his own character, as when he said that he had 'bedded every girl he wanted and some that he had not wanted' [Yalom and Yalom, 1971, p 487]. During these times, Hemingway was able to write and drink copiously during entire nights. He claimed to have written the short stories 'The Killers', 'Today Is Friday' and 'Ten Indians' (all published in 1927) in a single day: 'I had so much juice I thought maybe I was going crazy and I had about six other stories to write' [Oldsey, 1963, p 191]. He was also well known for his sudden spending sprees and his tendencies to fight[5]. Martin [2006] documented Hemingway's multiple references to suicide and mood swings in his correspondence. To his friend John Dos Passos, the writer confessed sometimes experiencing a 'gigantic bloody emptiness and nothingness'. He explicitly mentioned suicide in 1936, 25 years before he acted it out, in a letter to Archibald MacLeish: 'Me I like life very much. So much it will be a big disgust when have to shoot myself' [Baker, 1981, p 453; Martin, 2006, p 358]. Decreased libido frequently came in conversations and letters, as well as insomnia, and later on episodes of anorexia (Hemingway's weight varied widely across his life). These elements all lead to a diagnosis of major depression [Martin, 2006, p 354; Brian, 1988]. Such periods he called his 'black-ass moods' [Yalom and Yalom, 1971, p 493], and were likely worsened by the intake of reserpine [Little and Sharda, 2008], a treatment he was given for hypertension (likewise he took secobarbital, another depressant, to fight insomnia).

---

[5] Anecdotes are plenty. When challenged by Max Eastman with the famous line 'Come out from behind that false hair on your chest, Ernest. We all know you', he slapped him in the face with a book, and upon hearing of Eastman's later bragging of having thrown him over the desk, he offered the following statement: 'If Mr. Eastman takes his prowess seriously – if he has not, as it seems, gone in for fiction – then let him waive all medical rights and legal claims to damages, and I'll put USD 1,000 for any charity he favors or for himself. Then we'll go into a room (…) Well, the best man unlocks the door' [in Bruccoli, 1986, p 16].

The family history of mood disorders in the Hemingways is staggering, with 'a long history of affective disturbance, substance-related disorders, and suicide that preceded Ernest's birth, claimed at least three of the six siblings in his generation, and has continued on through two further generations' [Martin, 2006, p 353; see the Hemingway genogram in Jamison, 1996, p 229]. His father probably suffered from bipolar disorder. Maternal and paternal uncles also presented mood disorders. His sister Ursula and brother Leicester both committed suicide. His sister Marcelline was depression-prone, and conditions surrounding her death led some to suspect suicide (she also suffered from diabetes, like Ernest and Leicester, as well as their father). Hemingway's son Gregory, a doctor, was diagnosed with bipolar disorder, indulged in substance abuse and underwent sexual reassignment surgery after a lifetime of gender identity disorder (he lost his medical license and was arrested several times because of disordered conduct). Hemingway's grand-daughter, the daughter of his elder son Jack, also had multiple disorders, notably seizures, depression, eating disorders and alcoholism. She committed suicide in 1996. It seems reasonable to conclude that '[g]iven the family history, it seems likely that [Hemingway] had inherited a genetic predisposition for mood disorders' [Martin, 2006, p 354].

It is no secret that Hemingway was not always an easy person. He went through four marriages and his friendships were hardly stable. He was known for his tempers, sudden dismissal of previous acquaintances, and low threshold for irritation. Given the features of Hemingway's personality and relationships, Martin [2006, p 357] postulated the presence of a borderline personality disorder: 'In addition to the issues of identity disturbance and splitting, (…) difficulties with recurrent suicidal ideation, anger, impulsivity, affective instability, and unstable interpersonal relationships that characterize borderline personality traits seem identifiable in Hemingway's life story' [see also Brian, 1988]. Narcissism and self-absorption also seem a driving feature of his personality, affecting his relationships. He was often needlessly aggressive towards strangers and even his friends, often targeting their wives, who almost universally disliked him.

Although these observations are based on reasonable assessments of the available material, they cannot of course be considered definite diagnoses. What is more, as noted by Craig [1995, p 1073], the interactions or mutual exclusiveness of borderline personality disorder, major depression, and bipolar disorder are a matter of debate, as it is not clear whether these diagnoses exclude each other or represent variants along the same continuum [e.g. Gunderson and Phillips, 1991; Young, 2009].

Uncontroversial, however, was his well-known alcoholism. Hemingway drank in marked quantities since adolescence, sometimes supplementing any other nourishment for sustained amounts of time [Yalom and Yalom, 1971, p

492][6]. He eventually suffered from hepatic damage and was advised to stop drinking numerous times by physicians and friends, to no avail. From his war wound in 1918 onwards, almost each time Hemingway was hospitalized bottles of liquor were found in his room and even right under his bed. This is not to say that Hemingway was not worried by this state of affairs, especially in later years. He was nevertheless never able to sustain any significant period of sobriety. This dependence, of course, badly interacted with his already labile mood and could very well have led to brain damage, favoring the emergence of psychosis in his very last years [Martin, 2006].

In addition to these dismaying conditions and proclivities, Hemingway got involved in many situations were he suffered severe blows to the head. He was a lifelong risk-taker, avidly seeking danger in wars, bull races, hunting, boxing, and careless driving. During these activities, he clearly was reckless, often to the dismay of his comrades. He had many close encounters with death. In 1944, he was involved in a car accident in which he sustained a severe concussion. Three months later he had a motorcycle accident in France. On January 26, 1954, the Washington Post ran the enviable headline 'Hemingways survive two plane crackups'. This aspect of the writer's career is so central that Meyers [1987, pp 573–575] provided a detailed timeline dedicated to Hemingway's accidents and illnesses throughout his life in an appendix to his biography. To summarize, Hemingway went through several 'crashes resulting in brain concussions, hemorrhages, multiple fractures, severe cuts, and burns, and a lifetime of minor accidents, many associated with hunting, fishing, boxing, and skiing' [Yalom and Yalom, 1971, p 490][7].

As a result of his head blows, scalp lacerations, and skull fractures, Hemingway experienced headaches, temporary deafness, tinnitus, diplopia, slowed speech and memory difficulties [Martin, 2006, p 355]. Internal organs

---

[6] Anecdotes on his legendary drinking also abound. His close friend the Major General Charles T. Lanham recounts that when working on 'The Old Man and the Sea', Hemingway had the habit of swimming every morning in his pool until at 11 a.m., at which point 'his majordomo would come out of the house with what appeared to be a half-gallon pitcher of martinis', and the writer would then say 'what the hell, Buck, it's noon in Miami' [Yalom and Yalom, 1971, p 492].

[7] Although his temperament, risk-taking proneness and alcohol intake obviously contributed to his numerous accidents, an interesting alternative suggestion has been made: many of Hemingway's innumerable accidents might actually have been due to his poor sight. It seems that Hemingway was too proud to wear his glasses (just as he constantly struggled to hide his receding hairline), leading to many mishaps and involuntary blows to the head [Martin, 2006, p 357]. Nevertheless, this refreshingly cautious interpretation does not detract from the fact that Hemingway put himself in danger in many situations, all the more so by obstinately refusing to wear his glasses.

were also severely damaged by these events, further contributing to worsening his mood, and possibly precipitating psychosis and cognitive decline.

Hemochromatosis

A specific condition has been proposed as an overarching explanation for several of Hemingway's symptoms. This disease is hemochromatosis, sometimes also called 'bronze diabetes' or 'iron storage disease', an 'inherited metabolic disorder present from birth and causing an increased absorption of iron in the gut [as well as other organs]' [Beegel, 1998, p 375]. The evidence pointing to such an underlying disease – like most symptoms this article discusses – is mostly biographical. Hemochromatosis is rarely diagnosed before the patient is 50 or 60, as its symptoms tend to gradually increase in number and severity from the mid-30s onwards. The disease is an inherited condition of the autosomal recessive type, and its presentation varies greatly from patient to patient, depending of factors such as diet and alcohol intake. A diagnosis is normally based on the following triad: diabetes mellitus, cirrhosis of the liver, and abnormal skin pigmentation. Hemingway very likely had the first two, and the third one is difficult to assess due to his permanent tanning, as he was a man of the outdoors. There is also some evidence that his diabetes was inherited. Of course, cirrhosis of the liver is most often caused by alcoholism, but as Beegel [1998, p 377] explains: 'alcohol actually stimulates the body's absorption of iron, and because some alcoholic beverages (…) are rich in iron, a heavy drinker with hemochromatosis runs a far greater risk of developing cirrhosis of the liver than a non-drinker with iron storage disease'[8]. Male patients can also suffer from hypogonadism, due to iron-induced damage to the pituitary gland and ensuing hormonal disturbances. There are some indications that Hemingway suffered occasionally from impotence [Meyers, 1987, p 540], a symptom of hypogonadism, and this suggestion is further reinforced by the fact that Hemingway took pills of methyltestosterone in the 50s (which tellingly can induce depression, anxiety and insomnia, as well as hepatitis, all disorders from which Hemingway suffered at about the same period). Hemochromatosis, especially in the later stages, also has effects on behavior and brain functions, including memory loss, agitation, confusion, apathy and psychotic symptoms. The disease was never diagnosed as such in Hemingway, but was discussed by doctors during his stay at the Mayo Clinic in 1960 (they were however reluctant to perform the risky liver biopsy for confirmation). The writer himself became interested in medical textbooks about the liver, indicating that he had some idea

---

[8] Another argument against the primary influence of alcohol on Hemingway's ultimate demise is the fact that his father was a strict abstainer and nevertheless presented very similar medical and behavioral problems shortly before his own suicide [Beegel, 1998, p 382].

---

about the usual outcome of hemochromatosis (i.e. extremely painful terminal cancer of the liver).

The case for hemochromatosis is interesting but would obviously be more convincing if an official diagnosis had been made, in Hemingway himself or any of his relatives (no autopsy was performed after his suicide). The condition seems rare but probably remains underdiagnosed, as its features are often mistaken for primary ailments instead of symptoms of an underlying cause. As Beegel [1998] points out, the tragic irony of this state of affairs is that hemochromatosis, if detected early, can easily be controlled by regularly induced bleedings (this simple procedure allows avoiding the accumulation of excess iron). Moreover, an appropriate diet can also be recommended, as well as avoidance of alcohol. It is questionable, however, that such an early diagnosis and treatment in Hemingway would have 'enriched American literature' [Beegel, 1998, p 384].

In the light of recent developments, the hypothesis of an underlying hemochromatosis in Hemingway would also indicate the possibility of progressive cognitive impairment. Diabetes not only is a well-known risk factor for Alzheimer's disease (AD) and cerebrovascular disease, but also seems associated with mild cognitive impairment, a transitional stage between a normal cognition and AD [Luchsinger et al., 2007]. Moreover, the gene associated with hereditary hemochromatosis seems to be an additional risk factor for individuals predisposed to develop AD [Moalem et al., 2000], and there is some indication that AD might be associated with excess iron intake (as well as other neurological disorders such as restless leg syndrome) [Haba-Rubio et al., 2005].

Suicide

From 1954 onwards, Hemingway suffered a great deal from his accumulated injuries and ailments. His entire body was covered by scars, and he had problems in the head, heart, liver, back and circulatory system. The decline worsened markedly in the year 1959 [Meyers, 1987]. He could no longer fight or hide his depression and suicidal impulses. Writing became an ordeal, and almost all creative insight dried up. He developed psychotic delusions, mostly of the paranoid genre [Meyers, 1987, pp 540–544]. Most notably, he became convinced that some of his friends, the FBI, the IRS and the Immigration Bureau plotted against him. Ideas of reference were frequent, with an exaggerated tendency to interpret mundane events as directed at him. He also had delusions of poverty, despite his comfortable way of life. At about the same time, discouraged by the insults of life and aging, he presented signs of hypochondriasis: 'he magnified the significance of minor ailments and grew increasingly preoccupied with major ailments to the extent that his conscious thoughts, like the pages of his letters and the walls of his bathrooms, were plastered with meticulously kept charts of daily fluctuations in weight, blood pressure, blood sugar, and cholesterol' [Yalom and Yalom, 1971, p 493]. The etiology of these delusions is probably the long association of bipolar illness, alcoholism and multiple head trauma [Martin, 2006, p 359][9].

He was in such a poor shape that he accepted hospitalization on November 30, 1959, at the Mayo Clinic, in Rochester, Minnesota. There he underwent several courses of electro-convulsive therapy (ECT). Reserpine was discontinued as its depressant properties were recognized by then. However, according to Little and Sharda [2008], although 'his relapse and ultimate suicide occurred many months after the physiological effects of reserpine had abated (...), the protracted course of his depression and its damaging effects on his marriage, financial situation, and confidence in his ability to work might have been repairable at an earlier stage if reserpine had been discontinued sooner'. Of the ECT sessions, Hemingway wrote to his friend A.E. Hotchner: 'What is the sense of ruining my head and erasing my memory, which is my capital, and putting me out of business? It was a brilliant cure, but we lost the patient' [Meyers, 1987, p 550]. It is well established that ECT induces memory loss [Squire, 1977], but this is also the case for longstanding alcohol abuse, depression and head trauma. Nevertheless, it seems obvious that these sessions had a deleterious effect and might even have precipitated Hemingway's suicide [Meyers, 1987, pp 546–552].

The writer stayed 7 weeks at the clinic and was discharged after some (apparent) improvement. For some time, he could even write and was able to complete the memoir of his Paris years, 'A Moveable Feast' (published posthumously in 1964). However, what followed was a sad testimony of the depth of his despair. He relapsed into depression and became unable to write altogether. One day in April 1961, he was caught by his wife while loading a shotgun and had to be hospitalized again. Having asked to shortly return home to pick some items, he tried again to kill himself and had to be disarmed in extremis by hospital staff who were asked to look after him. He was then hospitalized again, but on his way to the Mayo Clinic, was seen walking dangerously towards a plane's spinning propellers. This gruesome attempt failed again as the pilot cut the engine. Having made 3 suicide attempts in 4 days, Hemingway was rehospitalized for 2 months. He underwent further sessions of ECT and returned home on June 26, 1961. There he still seemed to be delusional, as he claimed to see FBI agents monitoring him at a restaurant. Soon afterward, on Sunday, July 2, 1961, at 7 a.m., Hemingway shot

---

[9] A cautionary note is in order here, as it turns out that Hemingway was right about being shadowed by the FBI. The reasons are not entirely clear, but his affinities with the Castro regime and his acquaintances from the Loyalist Resistance of the Spanish Civil War might explain part of the authorities' interest in the writer. As Meyers [1987, p 543] put it: 'The FBI file on Hemingway proves that even paranoids have real enemies'. Likewise, his concerns about his finances and his health were far from entirely imaginary.

himself in the head. There is no doubt that he was extremely determined to take his own life. Shortly before his irreversible act he told Hotchner 'If I can't exist on my own terms, then existence is impossible (...) That is how I've lived, and that is how I *must* live – or not live' [Meyers, 1987, p 552].

Hardy and Cull [1988; Craig, 1995, p 1075] argued that the suicide was the 'result of draining vitality, proliferating health problems, increasing age, a declining ability to write creatively, and a diminishing sense of virility (...) combined with an increasing sense of despair'. Likewise, Meyers [1987, pp 558–559] wrote: 'the simple explanation is that he had a terrible combination of physical and mental illness that was caused by his neglect (even destruction) of his own health and that he had lost his memory during medical treatment at the Mayo. He suffered from weight loss, skin disease, alcoholism, failing eyesight, diabetes, suspected hemochromatosis, hepatitis, nephritis, hypertension and impotence. His body was in ruins, he dreaded a decline into invalidism and a lingering death'. Martin [2006] focused rather on the psychiatric side, pointing to the debilitating cognitive and affective effects of bipolar disorder, major depression, alcohol dependence, traumatic brain injury, and probable borderline personality disorder [for a cognitive model of suicide applicable to Hemingway, see Baumeister, 1990]. Finally, Beegel [1998, p 381], who defended the case for the hemochromatosis hypothesis, advanced the provocative idea that 'the belief, real or mistaken, that he was terminally ill may have contributed to Hemingway's suicide' (for a summary of Hemingway's ailments see table 2).

War Wound and 'Near-Death Experience'

We now turn to a specific event in Hemingway's life that several scholars have seen as a key element in determining his adult life and the contents of his works, namely the war wound he sustained during the World War I. At 18, Hemingway volunteered as an ambulance driver for the Red Cross on the Italian front. He came to Italy in June 1918, and then joined his unit in Schio, in the Dolomites. Having asked to get closer to combat zone, he was dispatched to the river Piave, where the Italians were busy stopping the advance of the Austrian soldiers. His duty there was to relieve the combatants by distributing chocolate, cigarettes and postcards. On July 8, 1918, at midnight, according to a Red Cross report, 'Hemingway was wounded by the explosion of a shell which landed about three feet from him, killing a soldier who stood between him and the point of explosion, and wounding others' [Meyers, 1987, p 30]. Hemingway recovered from the explosion and picked up a wounded soldier near him on his shoulders. But while trying to reach cover, he was hit again in the legs, this time by a machine gun. Incredibly, Hemingway would again stand on his feet and

Table 2. Psychiatric and medical factors contributing to Hemingway's affective and cognitive decline, and leading to suicide

Diagnoses	Description
Bipolar disorder	Probably inherited, widespread in family
Major depression episodes	Signs present at least since adolescence Depression worsened by reserpine and secobarbital intake (aimed at treating hypertension and insomnia) ECT treatment (inducing memory problems)
Alcoholism	Chronic since adolescence Liver failure, organic brain damage, withdrawal symptoms
PTSD	'War neurosis' Urge to revisit the traumatic event 'Near-death experience'
Multiple head trauma and accidents	Risk-taking Recklessness Poor sight?
Character problems Borderline personality disorder	Narcissism, aggressiveness, competitiveness, uncertain identity, difficult interpersonal relationships, need for adulation, depressive mood, need for excitement, fragile sense of self-worth, irritability, impulsivity, risk-taking and self-harm, suicidal Father's suicide. Anger towards mother and guilt
Insomnia	Associated with depression and alcohol intake, at least since 1926
Hemochromatosis	Diabetes Cirrhosis Dermatological disorders Cognitive, affective and behavioral disorders Hypogonadism, impotence
Psychosis	Delusion of persecution Delusion of poverty Hypochondriasis

bring to safety the wounded Italian soldier (who died soon after). For this act of bravery, he was awarded the Silver Medal (Medaglia d'Argento al Valore). The official citation stated: 'Gravely wounded by numerous pieces of shrapnel from an enemy shell, with an admirable spirit of brotherhood, before taking care of himself, he rendered generous assistance to the Italian soldiers more seriously wounded by the same explosion and did not allow himself to be carried elsewhere until after they had been evacuated' [Meyers, 1987, p 31].

He then spent 3 months in rehabilitation at the American Red Cross Hospital in Milan. There, he fell in love with an American nurse called Agnes von Kurowsky, who ultimately rejected him, adding an indelible psychological wound to his physical injuries. From the hospital, he sent a first letter to his parents on July 21, 1918. He then sent more details about the accident, on August 18, 1918, explaining that the '227 wounds (...) didn't hurt a bit at the time', which allowed him to walk '150 yards with a load' (the wounded Italian soldier), much to the amazement of his Captain [Baker, 1981, p 14].

Hemingway went on to say that it was only after he was carried on a stretcher to a distant station that his wounds began to hurt, 'like 227 little devils were driving nails into the raw' [Baker, 1981, p 15].

As the first American wounded in Italy, this event received some publicity in the New World, and Hemingway was invited to give talks. Speaking to a high school audience in 1919, he recounted the same event with some additions. We thus learn that for a moment Hemingway thought he was dead and 'moving somewhere in a sort of red din', but then felt himself 'pulling back to earth' and 'woke up' immediately afterwards [Bruccoli, 1986, p 4]. He also explained that he was actually, at this time, left for dead by the other soldiers, indicating that he seemed to be outwardly unconscious for some time.

A 'Near-Death Experience'?

This last account casually insinuates that something strange seemed to happen to Hemingway during the accident. He 'felt [himself] pulling back to earth' and then 'woke up'. Does this mean that at some point he felt himself 'out of earth', or flying 'in the air'? This possibility, strange as it seems, is quite likely. It has been defended most notably by Vardamis and Owens [1999], who argued that Hemingway underwent a so-called 'near-death experience' (NDE), broadly defined as a dissociated state of consciousness during a life-threatening danger. This concept has received (and still does) foremost attention in the occult literature and in parapsychological circles, as its most dramatic reports seem indicative, on the face of it, of a postmortem journey to an afterworld[10]. When introduced in 1975 to the general public, the NDE was described as a largely hypothetical

---

[10] Although the term was coined in a popular book fostering paranormal interpretations of the phenomenon [Moody, 1975], it must be noted that the term 'expérience de mort imminente' appeared much earlier under the pen of Victor Egger [1896a], a French philosopher who aptly predicted that these experiences would inevitably yield transcendental interpretations.

altered state of consciousness triggered by the proximity to death and comprising a number of dramatic features, including the experience of peace and calmness in the face of extreme distress, the feeling of occupying a disembodied and elevated perspective from which one sees one's surroundings as if 'from above' (including one's own body: out-of-body experience or OBE), the feeling of being propelled into a dark tunnel, the perception of a beautiful light, encounters with 'spirits' and 'divine agencies', a sudden and involuntary recall of one's entire life, and so forth [for reviews see Blanke and Dieguez, 2009; Holden et al., 2009].

To reinforce the hypothesis that Hemingway underwent such an experience, we reproduce two war NDEs reported in the literature (see below for Hemingway's own fictional accounts). Both individuals found themselves in bombardment zone, just like Hemingway [see also Vardamis and Owens, 1999, p 208]:

'A landing craft commander (…) was nearly killed when an enemy ammunition stock-pile blew up beside him [and felt] "as if I were sitting on a cloud looking down upon the whole scene, past, present, and future. Tremendous explosions were occurring all around me but faded and became a minor part of the whole experience"' [Noyes and Kletti, 1976, p 23].

'Instantly I was enveloped in a cloud of beautiful purple light and a mighty roaring sound (…) and then I was floating, as if in a flying dream, and watching my body, some dozen feet below, lifting off the sand and flopping back, face downwards. I only saw my own body (…) And then I was gliding horizontally in a tunnel (…) and at the end a circle of bright, pale prim-rose light. I was enjoying the sensation of weightless, painless flight but I remember saying to myself: "If this is death, it's rather dull". But I had a feeling it would be more interesting when I reached the light. (…) I became aware that I was being "sucked" back through the tunnel and then into a body that felt rather unpleasantly "heavy" (…) I seemed to have lost all sense of fear, but my back felt wet and slimy so I looked over my shoulder to investigate the cause. My back was a red mass of blood and raw flesh' [Fenwick and Fenwick, 1997, pp 43–44].

Although the NDE literature puts much emphasis on the similarities between these subjective experiences, there is as yet no workable definition of what exactly NDEs are supposed to be [Dieguez, 2008], and as these two accounts illustrate, there are ample variations from one report to the other (including the circumstances in which they occur, which sometimes are not life-threatening at all). More operational attempts have been made through the use of standardized questionnaires [Greyson, 1999], but these in turn, because they focus on very specific types of experiences, necessarily miss elements that might not fit one's idea of a 'prototypical' NDE. Therefore, claims that a 'typical NDE', or even a 'core NDE', exists, mostly beg the question. After all, the majority of experiences near death are unremarkable, as they merely involve unconsciousness or confusion. What is known, however, is that most elements comprising the general idea of an 'NDE' can be induced by a number of different circumstances (mystical states, mental disorder, substance abuse, epilepsy, stroke, deep or surface electrical stimulation of the brain, syncope, etc. [see reviews in Augustine, 2007; Blanke and Dieguez, 2009]), pointing to a variety of biological mechanisms.

Be that as it may, the most notable features to be found in Hemingway's account are the feeling of disembodiment (OBE), the conviction of being dead or about to die, the absence of pain, and the realization that death is nothing to be frightened of. The context in which the experience occurred and these features make it a classic case of 'depersonalization in response to life-threatening danger' [Noyes and Kletti, 1976]. Nevertheless, according to the scientific standards that were subsequently developed (and which are commonly used in current NDE research), Hemingway's accident would not unequivocally count as an 'NDE' stricto sensu for all researchers in the field.

Regardless of the definition of NDE one chooses to espouse, the phenomenon is still poorly understood. The problem, obviously, lies in the difficulties of studying in situ life-threatening events and the ethical obstacles in reproducing them experimentally (other ethical problems reside in the appropriateness of conducting parapsychologically oriented research in dying patients [Dieguez, 2009]). Nevertheless, a good amount of data, though most of it preliminary or somewhat contentious, is available on the topic. For instance, we know that OBEs are transcultural phenomena and that they seem related to some objective psychological and neural correlates [reviews in Murray, 2009]. Most recently, the OBE has been conceptualized as part of the more general category of autoscopic phenomena, namely experiences were a perception or a sensation of oneself in external space occurs, and related to a continuum of vestibular disturbances [Blanke et al., 2004; Lopez et al., 2008; Cheyne and Girard, 2009].

The description of transient analgesia, positive emotions, and paradoxical increase in mental quickness and physical strength during an extremely fearful or dangerous situation, has also been reported in the older [Heim, 1892; Egger, 1896a, b] and modern literature [Noyes and Kletti, 1976; Prince, 1982; Hood, 2007]. A classic example is Livingstone's account of having nearly died when a lion attacked him [McDermott, 1980] (see Appendix). These features strongly point to a sudden release of endorphins as a response to danger, inducing a 'limbic lobe syndrome' [Carr, 1981].

Pathological Influences on Hemingway's Works

Psychology and Psychiatry
In what follows, we examine attempts to link Hemingway's life, psychology and health to the contents of his works, most notably from the psychiatric side. We leave the effects of the 'NDE' for the following section.

Although the legitimacy of conducting retrospective pathobiographical analyses of works of art can be questioned, it seems reasonable to argue, as

Martin [2006, p 352] does, that in Hemingway's case at least this is 'an important task given the manner in which psychiatric disease affected the writer's life and informed his work, his writings being both products shaped in part by his painful internal mental states and defenses against them'. More simply, it has been said that 'no scholarly discussion of the author can ignore the man when attempting to analyze his literary creativity' [Craig, 1995, p 1059]. Such an approach is especially warranted for Hemingway as 'his material is psychologically, if not factually, personal: Hemingway's loves, needs, desires, conflicts, values, and fantasies swarm nakedly across the written page' [Yalom and Yalom, 1971, p 487]. Denying this in the case of Hemingway would take us back to the concept of 'the death of the author' [Barthes, 1984/1968], the contentious idea that works of literature have a life of their own, the 'author' being a mere 'scriptor' and his work becoming the sole property of the reader. In fact, Hemingway himself once wrote to a friend: 'good writing needs ideas derived from seeing life in arrangement, the design in life as it exists, not the trying to see life according to an idea' [Fuchs, 1965, p 437]. It thus seems inescapable that he would use his suffering and anxieties in his literature. Nevertheless, Evans [1961, p 606] warned that Hemingway's writings are 'more than a slightly fictionalized diary' and although it is incontrovertible that they represent 'to a large extent personalized fiction (…) the critic is dangerously myopic who sees in them only, or chiefly, the biographical element'[11].

It is indeed well known that Hemingway *fictionalized* his own life in his stories. An amusing example of Hemingway's embellished projections on his characters is composer Virgil Thomson's anecdote according to which 'while Hemingway in his Parisian years never bought anybody a drink, he paid them off in "The Sun Also Rises" (1926). He bought all his friends drinks in that book' [Monteiro, 1978, p 287]. More dramatically, in 'A Farewell to Arms' (1929), contrary to Hemingway's own experience, the nurse falls in love with the soldier, and dies in childbirth, which indicates the presence of 'fantasies of wish fulfillment and revenge' [Martin, 2006, p 359] in his works.

---

[11] To be entirely fair, the extent to which one should trust Hemingway's writings and claims as reliably autobiographical has also been challenged by the author himself: 'It is not un-natural that the best writers are liars. A major part of their trade is to lie or invent and they will lie when drunk, or to themselves, or to strangers. They often lie unconsciously and then remember their lies with deep remorse. If they knew all other writers were liars too it would cheer them up' [Bruccoli, 1986, p ix]. In an interview, when asked whether he sometimes wrote about situations of which he had no personal knowledge, he answered: 'That is a strange question. By personal knowledge do you mean carnal knowledge? In that case the answer is positive. A writer, if he is any good, does not describe. He invents or makes out of knowledge personal and impersonal and sometimes he seems to have unexplained knowledge which could come from forgotten racial or family experience' [Bruccoli, 1986, p 109].

We have described the Hemingway 'code hero' in the introduction, and in many respects this character is always Hemingway's idealized self, sometimes even too close to him to make a difference. Young [1966], who popularized the Hemingway theme of the 'code hero' (and summarized it as the tendency to pursue an unreachable ideal), described how Hemingway fully realized that what is important is the 'code' itself, not the goals it purports to attain, which often remain out of reach. This tendency is part of Hemingway's 'tragic vision of man' [Bruhans, 1960], and he seems to have projected it on his main characters and internalized it in developing his personal mythology. Like him, his heroes are psychologically and physically wounded, and strive to overcome even in the face of absurdity. Like him, his literary surrogates could drink all day long without being drunk. Like him, they have a tragic vision of life, mixing the utmost pessimism to generous vitality and heroism. Like him, they downplay their problems and carry on about their mission. Like him, they go to great lengths to test their limits, engaging in foreign wars, hunting in Africa, and boxing in or out of the ring. And like him, they are wary of women but ultimately cannot do without them. As a whole, his psychological buildup seemed to have been a force behind his creativity. Traits such as narcissism, competitiveness, courage, fierce independence, ambition, vanity, and grandiosity would eventually all coalesce to produce one of the most important and original writers of the 20th century.

It is well known that bipolar disorder can be associated with creative proclivities [Jamison, 1996]. Hemingway's spectacular writing output, sometimes completing several short stories in a matter of days and longer novels in a few weeks, was associated with a particular frame of mind that eluded him in darker periods of depression. He called these outbursts of energy 'juice'. Likewise, these periods prompted him to boast and display elements of grandiosity (see footnote 1). These feelings of self-worth, however, soon disappeared in moments of gloom. It is unfortunately impossible to provide a precise timetable comparing Hemingway's mood swings and his literary output, but we have seen that as depression and mental decline overtook him, his writing abilities declined.

Death, violence and suicide are themes prominent in all his works, from his earliest novels onwards. The suicide of his father was a major blow to Hemingway, and this event likely accounts for the widespread presence of weak fathers in his writings [Brenner, 1983]. This fascination with suicide, in retrospect, was a warning sign of the tragic ending. As Martin [2006, p 358] put it, 'The trouble is that Hemingway felt the need to discuss suicide in his letters to his friends at all'. This author even suggests that Hemingway's entire life, with its adventurous and risk-taking leanings, was akin to a continuous suicide attempt: 'he gave fate plenty of opportunity to do first what he eventually did himself' [Martin, 2006, p 358]. Therefore, the continuous presence of violence, injuries, killing and death in his stories can be interpreted as a function of an inner drive to project, control or simulate his own self-destructive tendencies. The fact that most of his characters, and their relatives, end up dying, likewise, is a strong hint that Hemingway saw no value in happy endings in real life either[12].

The majority of studies trying to link Hemingway's life and works are based on psychodynamic perspectives. Kubie, for instance, identified major themes of Hemingway's works as reflecting the fear of, fight against, and triumph over the fear of genital injury and violent death, and more generally fear of sex. Hemingway's insistence on masculinity, of course, was thought to combat the threat of passive homosexuality [Meyers, 1984]. The heroes of two major novels, Jack Barnes (The Sun Also Rises, 1926) and Lt. Henry (A Farewell to Arms, 1929), have been genitally wounded, and Nick Adams, in a number of short stories, is a typical wounded and rejected hero. Homosexuality and homophobia have also been perceived as recurrent underlying themes in Hemingway's writings, mostly because of the insistence on male comradeship. A collection of short stories was even named 'Men Without Women' (1927), making the topic of sexual identity an easy target for some critics [Drinnon, 1965; Brenner, 1983; Brian 1988].

A conclusion of Beegel's [1998, p 384] paper on Hemingway's hemochromatosis is that '[i]f his suicide was indeed precipitated by advanced iron storage disease, the unwary may find themselves unwittingly psychologizing an organic brain syndrome. (…) [T]he prevalence of a lack of passion, impotence, androgyny, and masculine overcompensation as themes in Hemingway's work, as well as his now celebrated "sexual confusion", may be more symptomatic of iron storage disease than of an overbearing mother'. Hemingway himself was indeed wary of the pitfalls of psychologizing, which in 'Death in the Afternoon' (1932) he called 'unavoidable mysticism', 'pseudo-scientific jargon' and 'pretty phallic images drawn in the manner of sentimental valentines' [Beegel, 1998, p 385]. Indeed, as Craig [1995, p 1066] pointed out, psychoanalytical approaches not only fail to explain how Hemingway's preoccupation with death, his alleged oedipal complex, and so forth, made him any different from all males, but also tend to ignore 'the role of [his] debilitating illness and physical disorders towards the end of his life, the role of medical treatment in the eventual outcome [i.e. reserpine], or the shock therapy that reinforced his delusions, the mental illness that plagued him at the moment of his death', to which we can add the brain damage induced by alcoholism and multiple head trauma.

---

[12] Hemingway was utterly dismayed by the happy ending of the Hollywood adaptation of 'The Snows of Kilimanjaro'.

Would an early diagnosis and treatment of hemochromatosis have 'enriched American literature', as Beegel [1998, p 384] suggests? This question can be answered by asking other similar questions: would Hemingway have been a better writer had he been treated for depression and bipolar disorder as soon as the first signs of his mood disorders appeared? Would American literature have been enriched had Hemingway been a fervent teetotaler? What if he had been more cautious, and avoided getting involved in wars and accidents? As one can see, the risk of retrospective diagnosis [Karenberg and Moog, 2004] is the temptation to rewrite history. The foremost characteristic of Hemingway, it seems uncontroversial to say, was his force of will [Donaldson, 1977]: 'Hemingway achieved what he did because he not only believed that he could do it but that he had the clear, hard will to carry it through. Indeed, so often over the years had will triumphed over the odds that only belatedly, and with stunning impact, did he recognize that some extreme situations could not be surmounted by that will. The clear and present signs of irreversible ageing and the unstoppable spread of disease, after his decades of overcoming physical injury of seemingly every form short of amputation, were not responsible to the will' [Monteiro, 1978, p 286]. Without physical and psychological obstacles, one's will cannot be put into practice and one cannot find out his true identity. Hemingway's life and stories never were about anything else.

'Near-Death Experience' and Art

Just like Hemingway's suicide does not need to be excessively 'psychologized', as he had plenty of physical problems, his 'NDE' certainly is devoid of any transcendental element, and does not warrant the kind of New Age interpretations the phenomenon generally receives from the media or most researchers in this field. In fact, Hemingway dealt with it as the down-to-earth man that he was, and never lapsed into the comforting spiritual overtones in which so many contemporary NDErs seem to indulge.

This is not to say that the accident did not have a profound effect on his life and works. This was his first real encounter with extreme danger and death; it served as a template for all his adventures to come. This early 'test' might help understand his fascination with danger and his need to display bravery in countless situations. Likewise, many scholars have speculated about the literary importance of Hemingway's war wound. Meyers [2006, p 30] merely says that it was 'a major turning point of his life', but others have drawn more specific conclusions. Most notably, Philip Young (the foremost biographer to have highlighted the importance of this event) wrote: 'The wounds in Italy are (...) climactic and central in the lives of Hemingway and all his personal protagonists' [Young, 1975, p 44]. The incident would have resulted not only in a 'castration anxiety', but also in so-called 'war (or traumatic) neurosis', which nowadays would be called post-traumatic stress disorder (PTSD; see footnote 3)[13]. Summarizing Young's thesis, Craig [1995, p 1062] wrote: 'Since 1924, Hemingway had been writing out the story of a hero that was based on Hemingway himself. It was the wound, the behavioral code, and the emotional adjustment required from these two issues that were at the heart of Hemingway's significant work'. The writer revisited this event and the very place in which it happened many times in his life and work, repetition being the hallmark not only of PTSD, but also of therapies against psychological trauma. He travelled back to the site of his injury, wrote about it in letters, talked about it to students and fictionalized it in a number of novels and stories[14]. In the words of Craig [1995, p 1063]: 'Hemingway's wound (…) was so traumatic that, through his subsequent works, he was continuously trying to work through the emotional trauma associated with his near death, returning to the scene of the injury by invoking the wound in his major works.' This 'repetition compulsion' has been highlighted as the key to understand the widespread theme of death in Hemingway's works [Oldsey, 1963, p 190]. According to Yalom and Yalom [1971, p 490], 'Hemingway speculated that the wound haunted him so because it punctured the myth of his personal immortality (…) [which was] no small loss, for an important premise of Hemingway's assumptive world was that he was markedly different from others: he boasted that he had an unusually indestructible body, an extra thickness of skull, and was not subject to the typical limitations of man'.

However, none of these authors has really discussed the particular phenomenological features of Hemingway's war experience. Without the OBE, perhaps Hemingway would not have focused so much on the events he suffered in 1918. An OBE is a highly memorable event, usually experiencers can recall it in vivid details and confer great significance to it, even long after it happened. Only Vardamis and Owens [1999] have paid close attention to Hemingway's NDE. Drawing on NDE research, they aimed at comparing two of Hemingway's works ('A Farewell to Arms' (1929) and 'The Snows of Kilimanjaro' (1936)) to the contents of contemporary NDEs. Although they acknowledge the highly speculative nature of their claims, they point out that even if it turned out that Hemingway never had an NDE, he was somehow able

---

[13] It is perhaps no surprise that Hemingway tried to block the publication of Young's work in the 1950s, just as he did for Kubie's paper in the 1940s (only published in Meyers [1984]).

[14] Most notably in 'A Farewell to Arms' (1929), 'Now I Lay Me' (1927), 'In Another Country' (1927), and 'A Way You'll Never Be' (1933).

---

to accurately describe in his work certain key details of the phenomenon that would be popularized only 50 years later in Moody's book 'Life After Life' [1975][15].

In 'A Farewell to Arms' (1929), the novel that launched his international success, Hemingway's own war wound is told through the words of the main character, Lt. Frederic Henry, who also felt himself rushing out of his body and floating in the air, all the while thinking he was dead, and then sliding back into his body and breathing again. The narrator also describes the state of shock of recovering and finding himself alive and injured.

The similarity of these fictional events to Hemingway's personal account in his letter to his parents from 1918 is striking, indicating that Hemingway had his own literary style well developed at only 19.

There are nevertheless dissimilarities between the fictional and the personal account. While the letter to his parents was meant to be reassuring and almost cheerful, as well as a rather objective description of the event, Frederic Henry's account does not hide the sense of angst and depersonalization that the event probably induced in the then young adventurer. With great perceptiveness, Daiches [1941, p 182] remarked that Hemingway did not write another novel for 8 years after 'A Farewell to Arms', as '[h]e was trying to find a world of intense living that would satisfy his personal tradition, and the novel was too rigid a form to be used for the recording of such a search'. The reason is that in 'A Farewell to Arms', '[v]ividness and intensity gave life meaning, and when these qualities departed, the meaning went out of life itself'.

The novel was written 10 years after the accident and, unlike the personal account, unambiguously reports the OBE. Although Lt. Henry is not Hemingway himself, the author later claimed that the fictionalized description was an accurate description of his own experience [Vardamis and Owens, 1999, p 209]. Moreover, in a short story anticipating 'A Farewell to Arms', the character Nick Adams, a wounded soldier, reports: 'I had been living for a long time with the knowledge that if I ever shut my eyes in the dark and let myself go, my soul would go out of my body. I had been that way (…) ever since I had been

---

[15] NDEs and OBEs can be found as literary ploys in a large array of literature, e.g. in Tolstoy's 'The Death of Ivan Ilych' [Haussamen, 2000], Wells' 'The Stolen Body', Kipling's 'At the End of the Passage'; London's 'The Star Rover'; Garland's 'The Coma'; Egan's 'Axiomatic'; Katz's 'Death Dreams'; Bishop's 'The Apparition'; Matheson's 'What Dreams May Come'; Shapiro's 'Simon's Soul'; and Werber's 'Les Thanatonautes'. Cinema also exploited the topic: Lado's 'La Corta Notte Delle Bambole di Vetro'; Schumacher's 'Flatliners', and Weir's 'Fearless'. Of course, the associated themes of the double and doppelgangers have also been much exploited in literature, e.g. by Oscar Wild, Guy de Maupassant, Edgar Allan Poe, Fyodor Dostoievsky, José Saramago, etc.

blown up at night and felt it go out of me and then come back' (Now I Lay Me, 1927).

More controversially, Vardamis and Owens [1999] also interpret 'The Snows of Kilimanjaro' (1936) as further evidence that Hemingway had an NDE and that it deeply influenced his writing[16]. However, 'The Snows of Kilimanjaro' is arguably the short story that yielded the most contradicting interpretations among critics [Evans, 1961]. It is a tale about wasted talent and remorse, the main character Harry, a writer, having 'destroyed his talent himself' because he let worldly pleasures turn him away from literature ever since he married a wealthy and controlling woman. As he is slowly dying from a gangrened leg in a remote African plain, Harry sees his past life in feverish flashes of memory. These memories are 'all scenes of action, contrasting by their very violence with the slow rot of which he is now dying, and they are connected with the vitality which has deserted him' [Evans, 1961, p 602][17]. Harry, in the company of his wife, is thus waiting for a plane to get him out of his misery. Death is approaching, as symbolized by vultures, a flickering candle and a feeling of oppression over his chest. However, 'suddenly it was all right and the weight went from his chest'. The next morning, the expected plane comes to rescue him. At this moment, the narration takes a strange turn: the plane flies over 'a pink sifting cloud', then through darkness and a storm, before reaching what appears to be the final destination, the Kilimanjaro, 'unbelievably white in the sun'.

What actually happened, unbeknownst to the reader until the conclusion of the story, is that this flight never took place. Harry simply died as he was losing his breath, precisely at the moment when 'suddenly it was all right'. Hemingway thus offered the reader a metaphoric and counter-intuitive final journey.

As one can imagine, the story has been interpreted in many different ways. For instance, it 'can be read as a writer's parable, a search for perfection in style and performance, with Kilimanjaro's peak a symbol of perfection' [Oldsey, 1963, p 188]. More generally, Hemingway seems to have depicted the quest for immortality, absolution, purity, permanence and idealism through artistic creation by highlighting the contrast between a wasted life and a glorious death, but also more pragmatically the deleterious nature of worldly pleasures and the

---

[16] This story has also been interpreted as a 'disguised representation of sleep paralysis' [Schneck, 1962].

[17] At the time of writing this story, Hemingway was, just like his character, in a period of slowed creativity, being married to a rich woman he did not love anymore and deeply anxious about having turned his back to his ideals of independence and his literary ambitions. Like Harry, Hemingway also had a bad journey in Africa, having suffered from severe dysentery and having been flown over the Kilimanjaro to reach a hospital. That was 2 years before he wrote the story.

---

dangers of women for the creative artist [Evans, 1961]. The success of the story itself represents Hemingway's return on the literary scene after some difficulties, as well as the beginning of a new life as he divorced from his wife and the bourgeois carelessness in which he indulged with her. Of course, the story is full of symbols, the most prominent being the peak of Kilimanjaro itself[18].

Vardamis and Owens [1999, p 211], however, interpret this allegorical account quite literally: 'In this story Hemingway describes the passage from life to death, not by delving into the realm of pure fantasy, but by utilizing real events and characters. The journey he describes corresponds to this aspect of the typical Near-Death Experience'. Through a convoluted web of associations, they argue that Harry's pilot in the story, Compton, is a representation of a dead person Hemingway once knew in real life, the pilot Denys Finch Hatton. This, they claim, shows that Hemingway 'anticipates the typical Near-Death Experience in which the "deceased" is guided into the afterlife by a friend who has already taken that path' [p 213]. They further argue that 'Harry's experience (…) bears close resemblance to factual accounts of Near-Death Experiences, which often include a life-review, a spectral guide, an out-of-body experience, a journey through rushing wind, from darkness to brilliant light, and, finally, a sensation of ineffable peace' [p 215]. Even if the OBE element does not seem present at all in this story, Vardamis and Owens manage to find one in the final scene, where Harry's wife, upon finding her husband dead in the morning 'represents Harry (Hemingway) detached from his body and looking down upon his own corpse' [p 215].

The final imaginary flight, nevertheless, is hard not to interpret in a religious or mythical perspective. For instance, one critic wrote: 'What Hemingway provides in a lay form of art is the mythic function of purity, of grace, of absolution – long a part of man's religious hopes. (…) In his imagined airplane flight he goes through death (…) and rebirth (…) to absolution to the House of God'. The same author then discusses the 'ascent of the soul, with the body left behind in the darkness of death' as an archetype of human mythology, and concludes that 'Hemingway was working out of an impulse toward purification and transference that has appealed to man so often as to have become an archetypical pattern' [Oldsey, 1963, pp 188–189; about the motif of flight and

---

[18] Here's what Hemingway answered to an interviewer asking him about his 'symbols': 'I suppose there are symbols since critics keep finding them. If you do not mind I dislike talking about them. It is hard enough to write books and stories without being asked to explain as well. Also it deprives the explainers of work. If five or six explainers can keep going why should I interfere with them? Read anything I write for the pleasure of reading it. Whatever else you find will be the measure of what you brought to the reading' [Bruccoli, 1986, p 120].

the ascending soul as a universal archetype, see Eliade, 1956; Pilch, 2005; Rock and Krippner, 2008].

The story has an overwhelming dream-like or hallucinatory character, as evidenced not only by its contents, but also by the writing itself, which uses loose associations and introduces some clever literary ploys such as italicizing the 'hallucinated' passages (except the 'final journey', which is written in plain text to enhance the illusion of reality). Bluefarb [1971, p 6] remarked that 'these scenes (…) [are] similar to the random thoughts of a patient under the influence of a hypnotic or sedational drug'. Varied drugs have indeed long been known to induce effects similar to 'NDEs' [De Quincey, 1971/1821; Sollier, 1896; Jansen, 1997]. Although Hemingway did *not* report a so-called 'panoramic life review' in the accounts we have of his accident, he nevertheless exploited the method of flashbacks on yet another occasion. In 'Across the River and Into the Trees' (1950), the main character, Colonel Richard Cantwell, proceeds to a 'voluntary life review' as he prepares to die, examining the main events of his life and the rightness of his past actions. This literary ploy reflects the constant sense of judgment that Hemingway applied to his own deeds, and does not seem to be associated to the typically *involuntary* 'life review' of NDEs [Egger, 1896a, b; Stevenson and Cook, 1995].

There are more obvious places to look for similarities with 'NDEs' in 'The Snows of Kilimanjaro' than in an allegorical 'flight' and a dubious 'panoramic life-review'. Indeed, the story begins with these words: 'The marvelous thing is that it's painless. That's how you know how it starts'. This sentence is strikingly reminiscent of a letter Hemingway sent to his parents on October 18, 1918, shortly after his 'NDE', where he explains that dying is 'quite the easiest thing [he] ever did', with slightly exalted overtones of his feelings of immortality [Baker, 1981, pp 18–19].

The absence of pain and realization that dying is an easy thing, as well as the personal conviction of being about to die[19] (or even already dead), are all processes sometimes reported by people who survive a life-threatening event [Sollier, 1896; Noyes and Kletti, 1976]. In this light, it is hard not to associate Hemingway's experience to the theme of 'grace under pressure'. Indeed, this is a motto that Hemingway marshaled from his early to his latest works. More than any mystical or transcendental epiphany, as is so often claimed in modern

---

[19] In an intriguing short story, Hemingway exploits such mistaken belief that one is about to die. In 'A Day's Wait' (1933), a young boy believes for an entire day and night that he is going to die because he misreads his temperature as 102° Celsius instead of Fahrenheit. In light of this story, it seems ironic that Hemingway himself would live up to read his own obituary in the newspapers on two occasions, once after a car accident and once after his two successive plane crashes.

writings on 'NDEs' (as far as we know, Hemingway did not find God nor a belief in the afterlife after his war injury), what the writer found instead after his war experience was his inimitable style as a storyteller and the insight to create his own mythological creature, the 'code hero'. The sudden reversal from fear and pain to peace and tranquility not only allows this hero to perform otherwise unimaginable skills, but more generally instils a feeling that one has full control over his own destiny. Anthropologist Raymond Prince [1982] called this situation the 'omnipotence maneuver', a term that would aptly fit both Hemingway and his heroes. It may be the case that the 'omnipotence maneuver' he experienced during the war remained deeply ingrained for the rest of his life and career. What few external observers could realize, however, is the tremendous pain and suffering that this 'maneuver' was designed to hide. The writer's final collapse indeed revealed the amount of energy needed to maintain the façade of self-worth that accompanied Hemingway throughout his adult life.

It is thus incontrovertible that Hemingway's war wound, if not his 'NDE', occupied a central part of his work and his outlook on life. In this respect, Hemingway seems comparable to other subjects who survived a life-threatening event, and who sometimes report a new outlook on life, feelings of immortality and invincibility, a sense of personal importance and a loss of the fear of death [Noyes, 1980]. Nevertheless, both the 'NDE' and the PTSD approach, though probably correctly underlying major themes of Hemingway's works (including some explicit references to war and wounds), should be more accurately perceived as additional factors to a preexisting personality pattern [Craig, 1995, p 1064]. Such a preexisting temperament might underlie both the selected literary topics *and* the very near-death experience. After all, it was certainly no happenstance that Hemingway would find himself on a battlefield in the first place. What is more, no single experience can produce good literature simply because it happened. For Hemingway, 'it is not the trauma but the use to which he put it which counts; he harnessed it and transformed it into art' [Young, 1966, p 71, quoted in Craig, 1995, p 1064].

Conclusion: Writing as Therapy?

We conclude by addressing the question of whether, considering the overall pathological picture we have drawn here, Hemingway developed his passion for writing as a form of self-medication. He himself answered in the positive. When asked to name his analyst, he once replied: 'Portable Corona No. 3' [Meyers, 1987, p 545]. In a short story, Nick Adams, Hemingway's favorite alter-ego, said: 'If he wrote it he could get rid of it (…) He had gotten rid of many things by writing them' [Young, 1975, p 39].

Critics also shared this opinion: 'Hemingway's writing can be seen as an adaptive defensive strategy for dealing with painful moods and suicidal impulses. (…) [He] may have told certain stories in order to ease the aches that life started in him' [Martin, 2006, p 359; Craig, 1995, p 1067]. For instance, we have seen how 'A Farewell to Arms' (1929) represents an almost explicit attempt to come to terms with his war wound and lost love on the Italian front (the episode is likewise revisited in 'A Moveable Feast' (1964) and 'Across the River and Into the Trees' (1950), and alternate endings to his failed love affair can be found in 'A Very Short Story' (1925), in 'The Snows of Kilimanjaro' (1936), and in 'The Sun Also Rises' (1926)). As Martin [2006, p 359] put it, 'twists of fantasy may have served as a defensive role for the author'. Actually, nearly all of Hemingway's alter egos in his writings are injured in some way (including Santiago in 'The Old Man and the Sea', who suffers from 'the cruelest injury of all – old age' [Yalom and Yalom, 1971, p 491]). In the end, however, the accumulation of repetitive traumatic brain injuries associated with mood disorder and alcohol abuse, ultimately leading to psychotic illness, 'would also have worked to rob him of one of his most adaptive defenses, his ability to write' [Martin, 2006, p 360].

Nevertheless, one can ask whether this constant revisiting and twisting of his own life really was of any therapeutic value. Hemingway aimed to control his own life, and in this sense, his creativity allowed him to successfully fix the failings of his real life. On the other hand, such behavior might be perceived as a form of denial, just like his reckless behavior in the face of danger. Such a strategy can only work so far. It is interesting to note that the only thing that Hemingway's characters did not reflect of his own life is his final suicide. Besides two hints at fathers' suicides (one in 'Hommage to Switzerland' (1933) and the other in the last of the Nick Adams short stories, 'Fathers and Sons' (1933)), none of his main characters commit suicide in his fiction. Yet, as we have seen, suicide was a constant feature of his adult life. In 'To Have and Have Not' (1937), Hemingway already wrote that all suicide methods have in common to 'end insomnia, terminate remorse, cure cancer, avoid bankruptcy, and blast an exit from intolerable positions by the pressure of a finger'. In the short story 'A Clean, Well-Lighted Place' (1926), we learn that an old man has recently attempted suicide, as a young bartender bluntly tells him 'You should have killed yourself last week…' However, we immediately learn that the old man is deaf. It took Hemingway 35 years after writing this story to finally hear the message in its cruelest intensity.

Despite the negative picture drawn here, it has to be highlighted that Hemingway displayed tremendous courage and resilience throughout his life, and it is no mystery that he became an example to follow for many American youths in his time, as well as a human and literary source of admiration for generations to come. In light of the psychological and physical burden he suffered, it might seem extraordinary that Hemingway managed at all to create such a number of acclaimed works. The fact is that despite all his flaws, Hemingway was a hard worker and knew the importance of discipline. With each new project, he embarked in what he called a 'training' period (inspired by boxing), where he would get into good physical shape, abstain from alcohol until noon and write steadily the entire morning [Yalom and Yalom, 1971, p 492]. And as Craig [1995, p 1079] notes, Hemingway was much of the time a very likable person, 'noted for his quick wit, perceptive observational powers, his enthusiasm, his magnanimous personality, his charm, confidence, generosity, and sentimentality as well as for his ambition and heroism'.

Like the protagonist of 'The Snows of Kilimanjaro' (1936), Hemingway sought immortality, or at least 'permanence in art form' [Oldsey, 1963, p 192]. He was certainly able to find it through his artistic legacy, as he seemed to be well aware when he wrote in 'Green Hills of Africa' (1935): 'A country, finally, erodes and the dust blows away, the people all die and none of them were of any importance permanently, except those who practiced the arts...'.

Acknowledgements

All Hemingway quotes cited in this chapter are reprinted with kind permission of Scribner, a Division of Simon & Schuster, Inc. and The Random House Group Ltd.

References

Hemingway's Works Mentioned (Chronological Order)
A Very Short Story (first published in 1925); in: The Complete Short Stories of Ernest Hemingway. New York, Simon & Schuster, 1987.
A Clean, Well-Lighted Place (first published in 1926); in: The Complete Short Stories of Ernest Hemingway. New York, Simon & Schuster, 1987.
The Sun Also Rises. New York, Charles Scribner's Sons, 1926.
The Killers (first published in 1927); in: The Complete Short Stories of Ernest Hemingway. New York, Simon & Schuster, 1987.
Today is Friday (first published in 1927); in: The Complete Short Stories of Ernest Hemingway. New York, Simon & Schuster, 1987.
Ten Indians (first published in 1927); in: The Complete Short Stories of Ernest Hemingway. New York, Simon & Schuster, 1987.
In Another Country (first published in 1927); in: The Complete Short Stories of Ernest Hemingway. New York, Simon & Schuster, 1987.
Men Without Women. New York, Charles Scribner's Sons, 1927.
Now I Lay Me (first published in 1927); in: The Complete Short Stories of Ernest Hemingway. New York, Simon & Schuster, 1987.
A Farewell to Arms. New York, Charles Scribner's Sons, 1929.
Death in the Afternoon. New York, Charles Scribner's Sons, 1932.

A Day's Wait (first published in 1933); in: The Complete Short Stories of Ernest Hemingway. New York, Simon & Schuster, 1987.
A Way You'll Never Be (first published in 1933); in: The Complete Short Stories of Ernest Hemingway. New York, Simon & Schuster, 1987.
Homage to Switzerland (first published in 1933); in: The Complete Short Stories of Ernest Hemingway. New York, Simon & Schuster, 1987.
Fathers and Sons (first published in 1933); in: The Complete Short Stories of Ernest Hemingway. New York, Simon & Schuster, 1987.
Green Hills of Africa. New York, Charles Scribner's Sons, 1935.
The Snows of Kilimanjaro (first published in 1936); in: The Complete Short Stories of Ernest Hemingway. New York, Simon & Schuster, 1987.
For Whom the Bell Tolls. New York, Charles Scribner's Sons, 1940.
Across the River and Into the Trees. New York, Charles Scribner's Sons, 1950.
The Old Man and the Sea. New York, Charles Scribner's Sons, 1952.
A Moveable Feast. New York, Charles Scribner's Sons, 1964.

General References
Augustine K: Psychophysiological and cultural correlates undermining a survivalist interpretation of near-death experiences. J Near Death Stud 2007;26:89–125.
Baker C: Ernest Hemingway: A Life Story. New York, Charles Scribner's Sons, 1969.
Baker C (ed): Ernest Hemingway: Selected Letters 1917–1961. New York, Charles Scribner's Son, 1981.
Barthes R: La mort de l'auteur; in Le bruissement de la langue: essais critiques IV. Paris, Seuil, 1984/1968, pp 63–69.
Baumeister RF: Suicide as escape from self. Psychol Rev 1990;97:90–113.
Beegel S: Hemingway and hemochromatosis; in Wagner-Martin L (ed): Hemingway: Seven Decades of Criticism. East Lansing, Michigan State University Press, 1998, pp 375–388.
Blanke O, Dieguez S: Leaving body and life behind: out-of-body and near-death experience; in Laureys S (ed): The Neurology of Consciousness. Amsterdam, Elsevier, 2009, pp 303–325.
Blanke O, Landis T, Spinelli L, Seeck M: Out-of-body experience and autoscopy of neurological origin. Brain 2004;127:243–258.
Bluefarb S: The search for the absolute in Hemingway's 'A Clean, Well-Lighted Place' and 'The Snows of Kilimanjaro'. Bull Rocky Mt Mod Lang Assoc 1971;25:3–9.
Bocaz SH: 'El Ingenioso Hidalgo Don Quijote de la Mancha' and 'The Old Man and the Sea': a study of the symbolic essence of man in Cervantes and Hemingway. Bull Rocky Mt Mod Lang Assoc 1971;25:49–54.
Brenner G: Concealments in Hemingway's works. Columbus, Ohio State University Press, 1983.
Brian D: The True Gen. New York, Grove Press, 1988.
Bruccoli MJ: Conversations with Ernest Hemingway. Jackson, University Press of Mississippi, 1986.
Burhans CS Jr: The Old Man and the Sea: Hemingway's tragic vision of man. Am Lit 1960;31:446–455.
Carr DB: Endorphins at the approach of death. Lancet 1981;317:390.
Cheyne JA, Girard TA: The body unbound: vestibular-motor hallucinations and out-of-body experiences. Cortex 2009;45:201–215.
Craig RJ: Contributions to psychohistory: XXIII. Hemingway 'analyzed'. Psychol Rep 1995;76:1059–1079.
De Quincey T: Confessions of an English Opium Eater. London, Penguin, 1971/1821.
Dieguez S: NDE redux. Skeptic 2008;14:42–43.
Dieguez S: NDE experiment: ethical concerns. Skeptical Inquirer 2009;33:44–48.
Donaldson S: By Force of Will: The Life and Art of Ernest Hemingway. New York, Viking Press, 1977.
Drinnon R: In the American heartland: Hemingway and death. Psychoanal Rev 1965;52:149–175.
Egger V: Le moi des mourants. Rev Philos France Étranger 1896a;46:26–38.
Egger V: Le moi des mourants: nouveaux faits. Rev Philos France Étranger 1896b;47:337–368.
Eliade M: Symbolisme du 'vol magique'. Numen 1956;3:1–13.

Evans O: 'The Snows of Kilimanjaro': a revaluation. PMLA 1961;76:601–607.

Fenwick P, Fenwick E: The Truth in the Light. New York, Berkley Books, 1997.

Fuchs D: Ernest Hemingway, literary critic. Am Lit 1965;36:431–451.

Goldberg M: On writing and publishing medical fiction. Ann Intern Med. 1997;127:413–415.

Greyson B: Defining near-death experiences. Mortality 1999;4:7–19.

Gunderson JG, Phillips KA: A current view of the interface between borderline personality disorder and depression. Am J Psychiatry 1991;142:277–288.

Gurko L: The achievement of Ernest Hemingway. College English 1952;13:368–375.

Haba-Rubio J, Staner L, Petiau C, Erb G, Schunck T, Machner JP: Restless legs syndrome and low brain iron levels in patients with haemochromatosis. J Neurol Neurosurg Psychiatry 2005;76:1009–1010.

Hardy R, Cull JG: Hemingway: A Psychological Portrait. New York, Irvington, 1967.

Haussamen B: Three fictional deaths compared with the near-death experience. J Near Death Stud 2000;19:91–102.

Heim A: Notizen über den Tod durch Absturz. Jahrbuch des Schweizer Alpenklub 1892;27:327–337.

Holden JM, Greyson B, James D: The Handbook of Near-Death Experiences: Thirty Years of Investigation. Santa Barbara, Praeger, 2009.

Hood RW Jr: Expériences de mort imminente due à des morsures de serpent dans un contexte religieux: une perspective jamesienne; in Brandt P-Y, Fournier C-A (eds): Fonctions psychologiques du religieux: cent ans après Varieties de William James. Genève, Labor et Fides, 2007, pp 19–43.

Hotchner AE: Papa Hemingway. New York, Random House, 1966.

Hovey RB: The Torrents of Spring: prefigurations in the early Hemingway. College English 1965;26:460–464.

Jamison KR: Touched with Fire: Manic-Depressive Illness and the Artistic Temperament. New York, Free Press, 1996.

Jansen KLR: The Ketamine model of the near-death experience: a central role for the N-methyl-D-aspartate receptor. J Near Death Stud 1997;16:5–24.

Karenberg A, Moog FP: Next emperor, please! No end to retrospective diagnostics. J Hist Neurosci 2004;13:143–149.

Little KY, Sharda AV: The vesicular monoamine transporter: basic and psychiatric aspects. Psychiatr Times 2008;25. Retrieved at: http://www.psychiatrictimes.com/display/article/10168/1153616?verify = 0#

Lopez C, Halje P, Blanke O: Body ownership and embodiment: vestibular and multisensory mechanisms. Neurophysiol Clin 2008;38:149–161.

Luchsinger JA, Reitz C, Patel B, Tang MX, Manly JJ, Mayeux R: Relation of diabetes to mild cognitive impairment. Arch Neurol 2007;64:570–575.

McDermott WV: Endorphins, I presume. Lancet 1980;316:1353.

Martin CD: Ernest Hemingway: a psychological autopsy of a suicide. Psychiatry 2006;69:351–361.

Meyers J: Lawrence Kubie's suppressed essay on Hemingway. American Imago 1984;41:1–18.

Meyers J: Hemingway: A Biography. London, Paladin, 1987.

Moalem S, Percy ME, Andrews DF, Kruck TP, Wong S, Dalton AJ, Mehta P, Fedor B, Warren AC: Are hereditary hemochromatosis mutations involved in Alzheimer disease? Am J Med Genet 2000;93:58–66.

Monteiro G: Hemingway's Hemingway. NOVEL: A Forum on Fiction 1978;11:286–288.

Moody R: Life After Life. New York, Bantam, 1975.

Murray CD (ed): Psychological Scientific Perspectives on Out-of-Body and Near-Death Experiences. New York, Nova, 2009.

Noyes R Jr, Kletti R: Depersonalization in the face of life-threatening danger: a description. Psychiatry 1976;39:19–27.

Noyes R: Attitude change following near-death experiences. Psychiatry 1980;43:234–242.

Oldsey B: The snows of Ernest Hemingway. Wis Stud Contemp Lit 1963;4:172–198.

Parker D: Profiles: the artist's reward. New Yorker 1929;5:28–31.

Pilch JJ: Holy men and their sky journey: a cross-cultural model. Biblic Theolog Bull 2005;35:106–111.

Prince R: Shamans and endorphins: hypotheses for a synthesis. Ethos 1982;10:409–423.

Rock AJ, Krippner S: Some rudimentary problems pertaining to the construction of an ontology and epistemology of shamanic journeying imagery. Int J Transpers Stud 2008;27:12–19.

Schneck JM: Disguised representation of sleep paralysis in Ernest Hemingway's The Snows of Kilimanjaro. JAMA 1962;182:318–320.

Sollier P: L'état mental des mourants [observations et documents]. Rev Philos France Étranger 1896;46:303–307.

Squire LR: ECT and memory loss. Am J Psychiatry 1977;134:997–1001.

Stevenson I, Cook EW: Involuntary memories during severe physical illness or injury. J Nerv Ment Dis 1995;183:452–458.

Trent B: Hemingway: could his suicide have been prevented? CMAJ 1986;135:933–934.

Vardamis AE, Owens JE: Ernest Hemingway and the near-death experience. J Med Humanit 1999;20:203–217.

Villard H, Nagel J: Hemingway in Love and War. Boston, Northeastern University Press, 1989.

Wilson E: Ernest Hemingway: gauge of morale. Atlantic 1939;164:36–46.

Yalom ID, Yalom M: Ernest Hemingway: a psychiatric view. Arch Gen Psychiatry 1971;24:485–494.

Young AH: Bipolar disorder: diagnostic conundrums and associated comorbidities. J Clin Psychiatry 2009;70:e26.

Young P: Ernest Hemingway: A Reconsideration. New York, Harbinger, 1966.

Young P: 'Big World Out There': The Nick Adams Stories; in Benson JJ (ed): The Short Stories of Ernest Hemingway: Critical Essays. Durham, Duke University Press, 1975, pp 29–45.

Appendix: Livingstone's Account of His 'Near-Death Experience'

'I heard a shout. Starting and looking half round, I saw the lion just in the act of springing upon me. I was on a little height; he caught my shoulder as he sprang and we both came to the ground below together. Growling horribly close to my ear, he shook me as a terrier does a rat. The shock produced a stupor similar to that which seems to be felt by a mouse after the first shake of a cat. It caused a sort of dreaminess in which there was no sense of pain nor feeling of terror, though quite conscious of all that was happening. It was like what patients partially under the influence of chloroform describe, who see all the operation but feel not the knife. This singular condition was not the result of any mental process. The shake annihilated fear, and allowed no sense of horror in looking round at the beast. The peculiar state is probably produced in all animals killed by carnivora; and if so, is a merciful provision by our benevolent Creator for lessening the pain of death' (from Livingstone D: Adventures and Discoveries in the Interior of Africa. Philadelphia, Hubbard Bros, 1872, p 15, quoted in [McDermott, 1980]).

Sebastian Dieguez
Laboratory of Cognitive Neuroscience, Brain-Mind Institute, Station 19
Ecole Polytechnique Fédérale de Lausanne
CH–1015 Lausanne (Switzerland)
Tel. +41 21 6931681, Fax +41 21 6931770, E-Mail sebastian.dieguez@epfl.ch

Bogousslavsky J, Hennerici MG, Bäzner H, Bassetti C (eds): Neurological Disorders in Famous Artists – Part 3. Front Neurol Neurosci. Basel, Karger, 2010, vol 27, pp 207–215

········ ············

'The Adventure': Charles-Ferdinand Ramuz's Extraordinary Stroke Diary[1]

J. Bogousslavsky

Center for Brain and Nervous System Disorders, and Neurorehabilitation Services, Genolier Swiss Medical Network, Clinique Valmont, Montreux, Switzerland

Abstract

The famous Swiss writer Charles-Ferdinand Ramuz suffered a stroke at 65 years, which he called 'the adventure' or 'the accident'. He developed language disturbances suggesting crossed aphasia in a right hander with left hemiparesis. This uncommon pattern allowed him to continue to write his diary and to report his disturbances, with a unique depth and precision, especially for cognitive-emotional changes. Language and motor dysfunction recovered within a few weeks, but Ramuz complained of persisting emotional flattening alternating with irritability, fatigue, depression, anxiety, and concentration difficulty, which gave him the feeling to have become another person and to be inhabited by a stranger, whom he compared with devils. Ramuz fought several months to resume his literary activity, having the impression to have lost inspiration and creativity. However, the novels he wrote less than 6 months after stroke show no stylistic changes and have been found to be of the same quality as his previous production. Ramuz even 'used' his stroke experience in his work, in particular in a novel depicting an old man who has a stroke and dies of it. Ramuz's diary, with his own daily description of stroke features and consequences during acute and recovery phases, is a unique document in a writer of his importance, and provides invaluable information on subjective emotional and cognitive experience of stroke.

Stroke is an extraordinary, traumatizing event, as reported by the patients themselves. For that reason, it is of particular interest to examine how artists and writers may have experienced a stroke, which often led to significant changes in their creative production [1]. Unfortunately, there have been only few writers who have written on their stroke. Charles Baudelaire developed aphasia, and could only reply 'crénom' ('damn') to verbal solicitations, while Valéry

---

[1] This article has originally been published in Eur Neurol 2009;61:138–142.

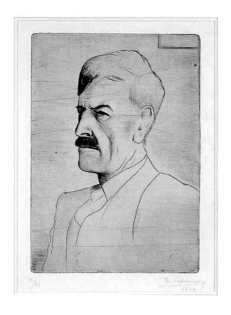

Fig. 1. Charles-Ferdinand Ramuz by Strawinsky's son Theodore in 1932 (etching, private collection).

Larbaud repeatedly muttered 'Bonsoir les choses d'ici-bas' ('Farewell, material things from this earth'), with no other verbal expression [2, 3]. One of the consequences may be the loss of literary creativity itself, especially when stroke is associated with aphasia.

By many, Charles-Ferdinand Ramuz (1878–1947) is considered the most prominent and famous Swiss novelist (fig. 1). In October 1943, he had a stroke with hemiparesis and language dysfunction, which slowly recovered over a few months. While biographers usually speak of a 'brain hemorrhage', it is likely that the stroke corresponded to infarction in the superficial territory of the right middle cerebral artery. We do not know in detail about Ramuz's risk factors, but he was a smoker (fig. 2). From the beginning, Ramuz was able to write down perceptions, feelings and remarks in his diary, and these pages probably constitute the most extraordinary literary report on suffering a stroke and recovering from it. The luck was that Ramuz, a right-hander, probably had crossed aphasia with left-sided weakness, so that he remained able to write normally with his right hand after language disturbances, which remained only moderate, had recovered.

Ramuz later introduced his own stroke experience in one of the novels he wrote only a few months after his stroke [4], which he initially entitled *Brain Shock,* before choosing *Accident,* and where he states: 'One says, an attack: I was struck with briskness … I was hit from behind, without having seen any-

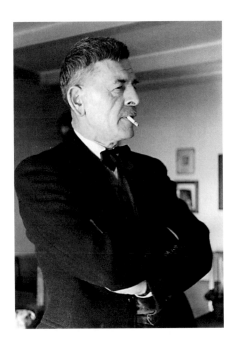

Fig. 2. Ramuz at his house 'La Muette' in 1941 (photograph by K. Businger, Fonds Ramuz/BCU-Lausanne, repr. L. Dubois, courtesy S. Petermann and D. Maggetti).

thing coming.' The recurring item throughout the unpublished drafts of that novel is the theme of a deep cut between before and after: 'There is on one hand the one I was and on the other hand the one I am now.'

Charles-Ferdinand Ramuz

Charles-Ferdinand Ramuz was born in Lausanne. He was given the first names of his 2 elder brothers who had died before he was born. After classical studies, he spent some time in Germany and in Paris, where he improved his literary production, focusing mainly on novels, after having also written poetry. After returning to Switzerland in 1914, he met Igor Strawinsky and Ernest Ansermet, with whom he created the famous musical play *Histoire du soldat* in 1918. Subsequently, his local literary activities, including a series of successful novels, made him become the most famous writer in French-speaking Switzerland. The novels focus on simple stories mainly from the countryside and peasants' lives, but with a very personal and sophisticated literary style, which made him the sole Swiss writer to enter (only in 2005) the 'Bibliothèque de la Pléiade', the Olympus of French literature publishing [5].

The 'Accident' or the 'Adventure'

These are the words used by Ramuz in his diary to name his stroke, which occurred between October 28 and November 3, 1943 [4] . Ramuz was admitted to hospital for several days, but unfortunately, no chart or clinical report has been retrieved. The first notes were written in bed on pieces of paper, which Ramuz subsequently pasted in his diary, probably without a reliable chronology. The examination of the actual diary shows that the writing was initially coarser, with a few phonemic paragraphias. Ramuz's first words already emphasized his efforts to recover ('to try to go back to life; to go ten times along the corridor and come back'), while the stroke itself is not really well detailed ['impression of imbalance (is it in my legs – or in my head)']. But Ramuz underlines a feeling of vital loss, which will accompany him for months, along with a loss of creativity: 'Everything is half dead in front of me, and I am only half alive.' Ramuz's description of the 'adventure' is very subtle: 'The adventure is sweetness … this is a caress but the result of the caress is the suppression of yourself or of a part of yourself. Something like the soft flight of a bat upon you, and then nothing will ever be the same.' He also reports an inner feeling of distortion: 'It seems to me that there is a transverse line from the right eye to the left hip, like these cards figures, and everything which is on one side of that line is more or less under influence, contrary to what is on the other side or above [.] One digests obliquely.' And this distortion leads to an inner dissociation: 'There is one part of me which is clashing against another one … [I am] excluded from myself.' This statement is reminiscent of what Ramuz wrote in *Histoire du soldat* 30 years before: 'You have no right to share what you are and what you were.' His immediate attempt to observe and analyze the effects of stroke is fascinating: 'I could have the opportunity to observe from the inside and to experience better certain phenomena, which doctors can study only from outside.' This ability to observe, analyze, and report in nearly any circumstance is typical of Ramuz, who immediately realized his fascinating, though critical, situation due to the stroke.

The 'Razor Blade'

This is how Ramuz described the acute stroke phase. He did not have many memories of the events which occurred during the acute phase, which he remembered as a 'darkening, out of which one finally gets out, but only to see that there is nothing in common between what one is and what one was'. This feeling made him think of 'the passage of [a] razor blade'. While Ramuz emphasized rather the emotional-cognitive changes than motor dysfunction, he immediately reported that 'the only external sign is this left hand; I cannot move the fingers separately. I cannot join the index finger with the thumb. I cannot bend the fingers against the palm of the hand. Arm atrophy … I can well hold an object, but I am forgetting what I am holding, so that it falls down, since the hand has no consciousness to hold it … I am aware to hold it, but there is no constant and spontaneous transmission from the center to the extremities.'

Ramuz developed left hemiparesis with brachial predominance. Three months after stroke, some degree of left hand motor dysfunction was still present. Ramuz reported that he was told that the left hand was moving as well as the right one, but he still felt quite disabled: 'I am thinking of that keyboard, where the keys just need to be so softly touched to say what they have to say; – what is true for fingers is true for everything. Pianissimos need all your strength.' Ramuz underscored his difficulties with the left hand, but did not mention facial weakness, while he mentioned gait problems only later. He never mentioned dysmetria or sensory or visual field dysfunction.

Aphasia and Cognitive Disorders

Witnesses and photographs show that Ramuz wrote with the right hand, and nothing suggests that he originally was a left-hander. Since he very clearly reported language dysfunction associated with left hemiparesis, it is likely that Ramuz had crossed aphasia. On the other hand, no usual right hemisphere syndrome was present (no anosognosia, hemineglect, or disorientation), suggesting that hemisphere lateralization of cognitive functions was largely inverted in his case. An advantage is that crossed aphasia is usually associated with good outcome [6].

Already in his first notes after the stroke, Ramuz reported language problems, mainly anomia: 'I have much difficulty in retrieving my words, even the most common ones.' His initial writing showed a coarser pattern with isolated phonemic paragraphias. He spent a night trying to 'reconstitute' poems by Rimbaud, Mallarmé and Verlaine, but the text seemed 'abominably mediocre', with changed meanings. He also reported reading difficulties, which suggested alexia: 'I noticed that I had problems reading and I first thought that my vision was weakened. I now see that this was not the problem, but something upon which it depends.' He also reported: 'some difficulty to read and assemble the letters, and then after assembling them, to go to the next line and put both lines together: and when this is a book, to know if what I am reading goes before or after what I have read: I mean, to organize the parts of a whole which I cannot capture, because the parts tend to exist only for themselves … a lot of words are missing.' Six months later, Ramuz still complained: 'I am eating my words; this is also happening while writing.' However, we have no document suggesting that he had coexisting agraphia. One month later, he noted: 'My love, oh! When can I start again? The words are pressing themselves from all sides against the walls of my skull, looking for a way that they cannot find.' In his novel *Accident,* which he started to write around that time, Ramuz mentioned the language disorder of the old Anselme, who 'was moving a thick tongue filling his mouth like with some sort of a cream, which precluded him to speak …, with sentences which he did not finish and with poorly pronounced words which did not follow each other.'

It is possible that certain difficulties with numbers, as well as other cognitive dysfunctions were initially present: 'some trouble reading time on my watch, the first days.' Ramuz also noticed that he could not adjust his tie, although his hand mobility was sufficient to allow it.

But what seems to have been especially prominent in the first weeks is a form of inner confusion, with difficulty in organizing his thoughts: 'I do not remember my novels characters [,] they have become strangers [;] my intentions have gone away, and what determines a style, the choice of words … I do not know anymore at which point I stand, but to leave things as they are, their disorder, this is still a witness of the problem.' Six months later, this problem was still present: '… loss of memory? I am losing myself into details. I do not know anymore what is to be written and what has already been written' (June 1944). In November 1944, over 12 months after the stroke, Ramuz was still complaining: 'Anything which I can still do is to wander in my room until giddiness, with an empty head. I am witnessing all this in a great chaos … my ideas have no more center, they are destroying each other. They are coming from where they want, they go where they want; I do not discern even the smallest reason why they arise.' These difficulties do not suggest memory dysfunction, but mainly an attentional disorder, which is typically associated with poststroke fatigue syndrome [7].

Emotional Disturbances

The study of emotional changes after stroke is rather recent [6], so that it is fascinating to observe how well Ramuz reported his own disturbances. Already in his first notes, Ramuz emphasized character changes: 'One is one thousand times more impressionable and irritable, so that one must soon become quite unbearable for surrounding people.' But Ramuz also found that there was some new sharpness in his feelings: 'Your inner reactions are much clearer about thousand questions that one can ask to oneself or that are coming from outside … what one would keep for oneself can now be expressed with violence and without care about oneself or others. And one gets some kind of enrichment of personality, at the very moment when it should have been damaged. What is difficult is that there is now a terrible exasperation of all inner moves, with such a violence that one cannot always control, and with particular angers … there are mood changes which correspond to total inversions of previous situations.' These remarks underline extraordinary observation abilities, but also unusual resources leading to new and 'enriched' emotional experiences, built upon the consequences of stroke.

Depression and emotional instability were mentioned early by Ramuz: 'and extreme depression follows the exaltation state … your life is divided into two parts while you do not even notice it … if one gets better this is only a remission.' On January 1944, the emotional imbalance was still prominent: 'and then this is an extreme irritability with violent angers about nothing.' Eight months later, Ramuz still found himself very fragile: 'I am afraid of everything. Much more than before.' He did not hesitate to use the term 'ruin' to describe his state: '<u>Ruin</u>. I am examining it to see what I can do with it … Now deprived of any pleasure: the sharp moments of joy which came about anything, and which were always leading to an inner awakening, which itself led to inspiration; nothing, a flower, a colour, on the wall, music, a bird song: well, now, I am insensitive to this: some sort of odd indifference to things and events … this is the finest part of my senses and of what feeling uses which has been damaged. No more direct contact: as if there was a very thin piece of silk paper between me and what I touch. It is sufficient for not perceiving with freshness.' In December 1944, over 1 year after stroke, anxiety remains prominent, probably more than depression: 'I am seeing with anxiety this being who has taken domicile in me, who is not me, who lives inside me, but who nevertheless communicates with the outside only through me, betraying me without cease … A being who obeys to only one feeling: fear; and even if I resist, it drags me into his own panics … A being who is like those devils in Holy Books, and whose lair is me …'

Ramuz's prestroke personality was not depressive or characterized by doubts as to his literary abilities [D. Maggetti, personal communication]. The poststroke emotional changes are thus even more striking, along with Ramuz's very critical judgment on his poststroke writings, while literary critics never made any comment on a possible 'change' in style or literary quality.

'Recovery' with a Feeling of Lost Creativity

Three months after stroke, Ramuz wrote that he had 'recovered', but that he felt deeply different than before the stroke, and he emphasized a sharp cut between who he had been before and who he now was: 'The adventure lasted two months. But what I am afraid of, now that it seems to have come to an end … is the impossibility to connect with my recent past, and to link me to myself … I am not dead, but this is my past which is dead.' A painful problem, which is not visible by other people, was a loss of literary inspiration: 'I am waiting for the impulsion. Will it come? I was still in bed when came a big surge for writing, but this is gone … I am now about like I was. I am well, I have no pain, what frightens me so much is the impossibility that I feel for resuming my work where I left it, and how little it interests me, and how much my thoughts of the time now have become strangers.' It is likely that mild cognitive and emotional impairment was sufficient to lead to this painful experience, while severer neurological dysfunction had disappeared. Ramuz felt changed and confused, and this compromised his desire to go back to writing: '… It is absurd to pretend to give an image of the world when one's own inner image is so confused. It is absurd to start with novel writing when this is so difficult to put things together. My mind is full of holes, which I am filling with great difficulty … I do not know what is missing … something in-between, certain intermediary reflexes, which normally are not conscious. Wait …' Although Ramuz restarted to write novels in spring 1944, he was still very unsatisfied with his writing 4 months later: 'I have lost my memory; and I cannot retrieve my words: this means (definitive?) inability to work. My attempts have been disastrous. Should I try again? Should I nevertheless, desperately, try to take advantage of my own destruction [?]' But writing remained a necessity for him: 'Write anything, but write. To force one's own hand to a mechanical movement. To put line under lines.' It is interesting that the novels written by Ramuz during that time are very similar to the ones he wrote before, and do not seem to convey a feeling of special difficulty or effort. However, Ramuz remained preoccupied with the image of a brain damage, as shown by a dream he reported 2 years later, in which an elderly man put a gun barrel to his head, and finally shot: Ramuz reported that he could feel very well the bullet 'progressing through his brain …'

It must be emphasized that Ramuz's literary style was not significantly modified after the stroke, as assessed by Ramuz's experts [D. Maggetti, personal communication]. No language disorder is noticeable, and the contrast between this absence of objective change and Ramuz's creative difficulties after the stroke is striking. A fascinating aspect is that as other writers or artists [1–3], Ramuz 'used' his stroke in his own creative work. These 'devils' who had taken domicile in him, as he complained, were eventually also the source of new experiences, feelings, and creativity, thanks to what indeed had been an 'adventure'.

Acknowledgement

I would like to thank Daniel Maggetti, director of the University of Lausanne Centre de Recherches des Lettres Romandes, for his encouragements, suggestions, and help.

References

1   Bogousslavsky J: Artistic creativity, style, and brain disorders. Eur Neurol 2005;54:103–111.
2   Bogousslavsky J, Boller F (eds): Neurological Disorders in Famous Artists. Front Neurol Neurosci. Basel, Karger, vol 19, 2005.
3   Bogousslavsky J, Hennerici M (eds): Neurological Disorders in Famous Artists – Part 2. Front Neurol Neurosci. Basel, Karger, vol 22, 2007.
4   Ramuz C-F: Oeuvres complètes, publiées sous la direction de Roger Francillon et Daniel Maggetti. Journal, tome 3 (1921–1947), et Nouvelles et Morceaux, tome 5 (1925–1947). Genève, Éditions Slatkine, 2005.
5   Ramuz C-F: Romans. Bibliothèque de la Pléiade. Paris, Gallimard, 2005.
6   Godefroy O, Bogousslavsky J: The Behavioural and Cognitive Neurology of Stroke. Cambridge, Cambridge University Press, 2007.
7   Staub F, Bogousslavsky J: Fatigue after stroke: a major but neglected issue. Cerebrovasc Dis 2001;12:75–81.

Julien Bogousslavsky, MD
Center for Brain and Nervous System Disorders, and Neurorehabilitation Services
Genolier Swiss Medical Network, Clinique Valmont
CH–1823 Glion/Montreux (Switzerland)
Tel. +41 21 962 3700, Fax +41 21 962 3838, E-Mail jbogousslavsky@valmontgenolier.ch

Bogousslavsky J, Hennerici MG, Bäzner H, Bassetti C (eds): Neurological Disorders in Famous
Artists – Part 3. Front Neurol Neurosci. Basel, Karger, 2010, vol 27, pp 216–226

....

Portrayal of Neurological Illness and Physicians in the Works of Shakespeare

Brandy R. Matthews

Indiana University School of Medicine, Indiana Alzheimer Disease Center,
Indianapolis, Ind., USA

Abstract

William Shakespeare was arguably one of the most prolific writers of all time. The topics explored in his works include both physicians and neurological illnesses. In addition to a
review of the portrayal of neurological diseases such as dementia, epilepsy, parkinsonism,
and parasomnias, this article describes the roles of physicians in Shakespeare's plays.
Furthermore, a novel hypothesis that King Lear, one of Shakespeare's more tragic figures,
suffered from dementia with Lewy bodies is explored based on evidence from the dialogue
of the drama.

...his...brain – Which some suppose the soul's frail dwelling-house...
King John V.vii.2–3

Shakespeare on Neurological Conditions

William Shakespeare (fig. 1), born in 1564 at Stratford-upon-Avon,
England, was arguably the most eminent and prolific writer in recorded history.
Credited with 37 plays and 154 sonnets, his extensive collection of timeless
tales is unrivalled, even engendering doubt as to the feasibility of a minimally
educated actor producing so many works of brilliance during his 52 years of
life [Murray, 2003]. Controversies aside, he was recently voted 'Man of the
Millennium', reflecting his persistent influence on Western culture. His plays
continue to be produced throughout the world and have spawned over 300 television and film versions with many other modern adaptations [Peacock, 2002].
Although Shakespeare attended grammar school, he did not attend university,

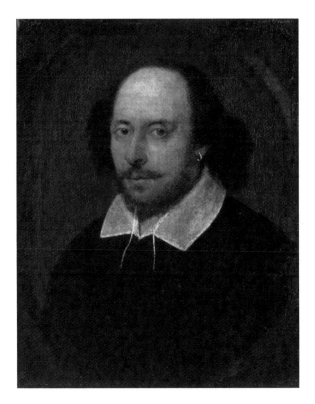

Fig. 1. William Shakespeare attributed to John Taylor. ©National Portrait Gallery, London, UK. Reproduced with kind permission.

but this lack of formal, higher education did not prevent the Bard from developing uncanny powers of observation. His eerily accurate portrayal of medical and psychiatric illness has led some to speculate that he frequented the insane asylum at Bethlehem ('Bedlam') [Andreasen, 1976] or, later in his career, consulted with his daughter's husband, Dr. John Hall [Peacock, 2002]. In any case, without medical training, Shakespeare described various neurological disorders with keen insight. He demonstrated awareness of not only signs and symptoms, but, perhaps more importantly for a dramatist, the broader consequences for the afflicted and caregivers, including physicians. While several lines make negative reference to the medical profession, overall the portrayal of physicians in Shakespeare's plays is favorable. Although none of the physicians is specifically identified as a neurologist, it is clear that the master playwright was intrigued by the function of the human brain.

Several neurological conditions which appear in the works of Shakespeare have been the topic of previous discussion in the medical literature (selected examples are provided in table 1, along with appropriate dialogue and references.) Epilepsy is the neurological illness portrayed most frequently with two of Shakespeare's plays including an irrefutable description of seizures [Fogan, 1989]. In *Julius Caesar*, Cassius refers to the title character when he reports:

And, when the fit was on him, I did mark
How he did shake: 'tis true, this god did shake:
His coward lips did from their colour fly;
And that same eye, whose bend doth awe the world,
Did lose his luster: I did hear him groan:
Ay, and that tongue of his… (*I.ii*.120–125)

Later, Casca proclaims, 'He fell down in the market-place, and foam'd at the mouth, and was speechless' (*I.ii*.252–253). *Othello* includes a seizure witnessed on the stage which is preceded by disorganized mumbling voiced by the title character, presumably representing an aura [Kail, 1986]. The treacherous Iago has observed a seizure cluster and gives the following foreshadowing commentary during the episode:

My lord is fall'n into an epilepsy:
This is his second fit; he had one yesterday…
The lethargy must have his quiet course:
If not he foams at mouth, and by and by
Breaks out to savage madness (*IV.i*.50–55).

Less specific references to 'fits' are made in *Macbeth* and *King Henry IV, part 2*. Lady Macbeth informs her guests of what may represent an absence seizure:

…My lord is often thus,
And hath been from his youth. Pray you, keep seat.
The fit is momentary; upon a thought
He will again be well… (*III.iv*.53–56).

While Warwick advises King Henry's Princes, 'Be patient, Princes; you do know these fits/ Are with his highness very ordinary' (*IV.iv*.114–115). Another epilepsy reference occurs in *King Lear* when Kent shouts to the unliked Oswald, 'A plague upon your epileptic visage' (*II.ii*.78). It is notable that Shakespeare's portrayal of epilepsy is compassionate by the standards of the day, when seizures were likened to witchcraft [Kail, 1986].

Modern Interpretation of the Neurological Illness of King Lear

The cognitive and emotional symptoms demonstrated by the elderly King Lear have been the topic of several psychiatric case discussions (fig. 2).

Table 1. Neurological illness in the works of William Shakespeare

Neurological diagnosis	Shakespearian play	Character affected	Selected dialogue evidence[1]	Selected references
Dementia	*King Lear*	King Lear	'Where have I been? Where am I?…I am a very foolish, fond old man,/ Fourscore and upward… I fear I am not in my perfect mind./ Methinks I should know you…yet, I am doubtful: for I am mainly ignorant/ What place this is; and all the skill I have/ Remembers not these garments; nor I know not/ Where I did lodge last night.' *IV.vii.51–67*	Andreasen, 1976; Fogan, 1989; Kail, 1986
Dementia	*Winter's Tale*	Florizel's father (as described by Polixenes)	'Is not your father grown incapable/ Of reasonable affairs? Is he not stupid/ With age and alt'ring rheums? can he speak? hear?/ Know man from man? Dispute his own estate?/ Lies he not bed-rid? And again does nothing/ But what he did being childish?' *IV.iii.401–406*	Fogan, 1989
Epilepsy	*Othello*	Othello	'My lord is fall'n into an epilepsy. This is his second fit…The lethargy must have his quiet course; If not he foams at mouth, and by and by/ Breaks out to savage madness.' *IV.i.50–55*	Fogan, 1989
Epilepsy	*Julius Caesar*	Julius Caesar	'And when the fit was on him I did mark/ How he did shake.' *I.ii.120.* 'He fell down in the market-place, and foam'd at the mouth, and was speechless.' *I.ii.252–253*	Fogan, 1989; Kail, 1986
Epilepsy	*Macbeth*	Macbeth	'Then comes my fit again.' *III.iv.21*	Kail, 1986
Epilepsy	*King Lear*	Oswald	'A plague upon your epileptic visage.' *II.ii.78*	Kail, 1986

Table 1. (continued)

Neurological diagnosis	Shakespearian play	Character affected	Selected dialogue evidence[1]	Selected references
Parasomnia	*Macbeth*	Lady Macbeth	'I have seen/ her rise from her bed, throw her nightgown upon/ her, unlock her closet, take forth paper, fold it,/ write upon't, read it, afterwards seal it, and again/ return to bed; yet all this while in the most fast/ sleep.' *V.i.4–9*	Fogan, 1989; Furman et al, 1997
Parkinsonism	*Troilus and Cressida*	Achilles	'…the faint defects of age/… to cough and spit,/ And with a palsy fumbling on his gorget,/ Shake in and out the rivet…' *I.iii.172–175*	Stein, 2005
Prion disease	*Macbeth*	Macbeth	'Round about the cauldron go/ In the poison'd entrails throw.' *IV.i.4–5* 'Ere, we will eat our meal in fear…' *III.ii.17.* 'I have a strange infirmity…' *III.iv.85*	Norton et al, 2006
Scoliosis/ brachial plexus injury	*King Henry VI, part 3*; *King Richard III*	Richard III	'…She did corrupt frail nature with some bribe,/ To shrink mine arm up like a wither'd shrub;/ To make an envious mountain on my back,/ Where sits deformity to mock my body;/ To shape my legs of an unequal size,/ To disproportion me in every part…' *King Henry VI, part 3 III.ii.155–160* '…behold, mine arm/ Is, like a blasted sapling, wither'd up…' *King Richard III III.iv.69–70*	Fogan, 1989
Sleep apnea	*King Henry IV*	Falstaff	'Falstaff!–fast asleep…and snorting like a horse. / Hark, how hard he fetches breath.' *II.iv.543–545*	Furman et al, 1997; Adler,1983

Table 1. (continued)

Neurological diagnosis	Shakespearian play	Character affected	Selected dialogue evidence[1]	Selected references
Stroke/seizure	*King Henry IV, part 2*	King Henry IV	'…his highness is faln into… apoplexy…a kind of lethargy… a kind of sleeping in the blood …it hath its original from… perturbation of the brain…' *I. ii.110–119*	Fogan, 1989; Kail, 1986
Tremor	*King Henry VI, part 2*	Lord Say	'Why dost thou quiver, man?/ It is the palsy, and not fear, provokes me.' *IV.vii.90–91* "…he nods at us…I'll see if his head will stand steadier on a pole." *IV.vii.92–94*	Fogan, 1989; Stein, 2005

[1] All quotations from the various works of William Shakespeare cited are referenced by play, act, scene, and line(s) in an effort to facilitate cross-referencing with other published versions. All citations herein were taken from: William Shakespeare: The Complete Works. New York, Barnes & Noble, 1994.

Although Sigmund Freud is likely the most notorious clinician to write about *King Lear*, other discerning commentaries from the 18th century and beyond have been offered by prominent clinicians in psychiatry including Brigham and Ray [Edgar, 1961]. The diagnoses rendered have been diverse including: organic brain syndrome, mania, depression, delirium, reactive psychosis, and bipolar disorder [Andreasen, 1976; Truskinovsky, 2002]. This differential is conceivable in the context of the play's action as the King proclaims, '…the tempest in my mind,/Doth from my senses take all feelings else,/Save what beats there' *(III.iv.57–59)*. However, diagnostic considerations in this case have expanded with current understanding in neurodegenerative disease, and therefore warrant additional exploration.

Briefly, at the center of the play's complex action Lear, the aging King of Britain, determines to split his domain amongst his three daughters. Goneril and Regan, gush and flatter, but Cordelia with characteristic integrity refuses to be party to her father's whims. As a consequence, she is promptly disinherited, and as disguised misadventures ensue, the King's mental status declines when he discovers the realities of his family situation. While some have concurred with Shakespeare's dialogue, ''Tis the infirmity of his age…' *(I.i.94)*, to suggest that the decline in Lear's ability to reason is a reflection of advancing age

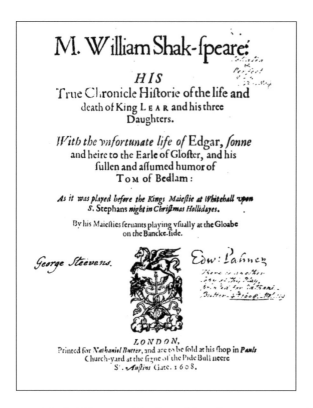

Fig. 2. Title page of the first edition of *King Lear* (1608) by William Shakespeare. The handwritten words are the signatures of the book's various owners.

and 'senile dementia' [Fogan,1989; Kail, 1986], modern neurologists and many laypersons recognize that signs and symptoms of dementia are not a necessary consequence of aging [Anstey and Low, 2004; Hawley et al., 2006]. Authors maintaining that Lear suffered from a psychiatric illness rather than a neurodegenerative disorder counter that lucid intervals, maintained physical fitness, and an ability to clearly recollect all of his daughters' presumed past and present offenses, render a diagnosis of dementia unlikely [Truskinovsky, 2002].

The cited lucid intervals may alternatively be described as fluctuations in cognition which may herald delirium in King Lear, as advanced by Donnelly [1953]; however, this symptom also represents one of the core features of dementia with Lewy bodies (DLB). Further investigation into the text of the play and comparison with the revised criteria for the diagnosis of DLB [McKeith et al., 2005] render a posthumous diagnosis of probable DLB tenable in the case of King Lear.

Regarding the central feature of DLB, King Lear clearly demonstrates cognitive decline which results in occupational dysfunction in the play's opening scene when he opts to divide his country and give up the role of governance in exchange for the forced flattery of his daughters. The disastrous consequences of King Lear's social dysfunction as related to his family are evidenced in the same scene during this irrational exchange when the King disinherits Cordelia:

> *King Lear*: Which of you shall we say dost love us most?…
> …Speak…
> *Cordelia*: Unhappy that I am, I cannot heave
> My heart into my mouth: I love you majesty
> According to my bond; no more or less…
> *King Lear*: …Here I disclaim all my paternal care,
> Propinquity and property of blood,
> And as a stranger to my heart and me
> Hold thee, from this, for ever… *(I.i.51–116)*

Of the DLB core features, there is evidence to support the presence of all three in King Lear's case. Cognitive fluctuation is well demonstrated in adjacent speeches in Act IV, when King Lear initially rambles incoherently (while also describing another core feature: visual hallucinations), then demonstrates profound clarity in describing his situation to the Earl of Gloster:

> Nature's above art in that respect. – There's your
> press-money. That fellow handles his bow like a
> crow-keeper: draw me a clothier's yard. – Look,
> look, a mouse! Peace, peace; – this piece of
> toasted cheese will do't. – There's my gauntlet;
> I'll prove it on a giant. – Bring up the brown bills.
> – O, wellflown, bird! – I'the clout, I'the clout:
> Hewgh! – Give the word…
> …They flattered
> me like a dog; and told me I had white hairs
> in my beard ere the black ones were there. – To
> say 'ay' and 'no' to everything that I said!…
> …they told me
> I was everything; 'tis a lie… *(IV.vi.86–106)*

Regarding a third core feature of DLB, spontaneous features of parkinsonism, at least two possible signs of parkinsonism emerge in the action of the play. Hypokinetic speech may be represented by Shakespeare's departure from standard iambic pentameter in many of King Lear's speeches, using the poetic devices of enjambment and pyrrhic feet to increase the speed and urgency of line recitation. While these techniques have previously been cited as evidence of pressured speech [Truskinovsky, 2002], the outcome is equally consistent with hypokinetic dysarthria associated with basal ganglia disease. Subtle fine motor dysfunction may also be evidenced by the King's request, 'Pray you, undo this button' *(V.iii.114)*.

In addition to the visual hallucinations described above, King Lear also had systematized delusions, a supportive feature in DLB, as exemplified by imagining the Fool to be a noble philosopher in Act III. He may have experienced delusional misidentification during the following encounter with Cordelia:

> You are a spirit, I know…
> I fear I am not in my perfect mind.
> Methinks I should know you…
> Yet I am doubtful…
> For, as I am a man, I think this lady
> To be my child Cordelia. *(IV.vii.48–70)*

Other supportive features represented in the play include tactile hallucinations (i.e. '…mine own tears/Do scald like molten lead' *(IV.vii.46–47)*) and depression (i.e. 'If you have poison for me, I will drink it' *(IV.vii.72)*).

One need not ignore the themes of pride, trust, and integrity revealed in Shakespeare's complex character, King Lear, to take comfort in the fact that many of the King's probable DLB symptoms would have responded to modern medications such as cholinesterase inhibitors, antidepressants, and atypical antipsychotics [McKeith et al., 2005]. Avoiding anachronism, King Lear's doctor was without adequate therapy and could offer only the following consolation to Cordelia, 'Be comforted, good madam: the great rage,/You see, is kill'd in him…' *(IV.vii.78)*.

Shakespeare's Physicians

Shakespeare's plays give rise to 8 physicians as characters and countless other references to doctors and medicine [Kail, 1983, 1990]. Unfortunately, a portion of these references are not favorable; some are nearly as inflammatory as the oft-quoted line in *King Henry VI, part 2,* 'First thing we do, let's kill all the lawyers' *(IV.ii.74)*. In *King Lear,* the Earl of Kent exclaims, 'Kill thy physician, and the fee bestow upon the foul disease' *(I.ii.165–166)*. The only onstage doctor who gives rise to ridicule is Doctor Caius in *The Merry Wives of Windsor*:

> He has no more knowledge of Hibbocrates [sic] and
> Galen, – and he is a knave besides; a cowardly
> Knave as you would desires to be acquainted
> Withal. *(III.i.63–66)*

Representing more admirable traits, the Scottish physician intrigued by the somnambulism and somniloquy of Lady Macbeth demonstrates humility and wisdom in the following exchange with the volatile *Macbeth*:

Macbeth: Cure her of that:
Cans't thou not minister to a mind diseased;
Pluck from the memory a rooted sorrow,
Raze out the written troubles of the brain,
And with some sweet oblivious antidote
Cleanse the stuft bosom of that perilous stuff
Which weighs upon the heart?
Doctor: …therein the patient
Must minister to himself. *(V.iii.39–46)*

Perhaps the greatest tribute to physicians in the works of Shakespeare is spoken in *Pericles* by Cerimon, who some believe to be modeled after the Bard's son-in-law [Kail, 1983, 1990]:

I hold it ever,
Virtue and cunning were endowments greater
Than nobleness and riches…
…I have –
Together with my practice – made familiar
To me and to my aid the blest infusions
That dwell in vegetives, in metals, stones;
And I can speak of the disturbances
That nature works, and of her cures; which doth give me
A more content in course of true delight
Than to be thirsty after tottering honour… *(III.ii.26–40)*

Shakespeare Therapy?

If Shakespeare's empathic and complex portrayal of those suffering from neurological illness and of the physicians who offer them care is a reflection of his own character, then he would surely be pleased to realize that his dramas are now being used 'therapeutically'. For example, two recent documentary films strive to reveal the healing power of his plays. In Mel Stuart's 2004 'The Hobart Shakespeareans', Rafe Esquith, a teacher in central Los Angeles, Calif., encourages his elementary school students to escape the poverty and violence of their community by dedicating their efforts to an awe-inspiring performance of *Hamlet*. Hank Rogerson and Jilann Spitzmiller's 'Shakespeare Behind Bars' (2005) likewise explores the themes of redemption and forgiveness as prisoners in a southern United States maximum security prison commit to understanding and performing *The Tempest*. Such updated celebrations of Shakespeare as master creator and captivator of humanity resound with hope for the future, echoing his own words: *All's Well that Ends Well*!

Acknowledgements

This work was originally presented as a seminar at the American Academy of Neurology Annual Meeting 2007, Boston, Mass., USA, and is reproduced here with full permission. All quotations from the various works of William Shakespeare cited within this text are referenced by play, act, scene, and line(s) in an effort to facilitate cross-referencing with other published versions. All citations herein were taken from: William Shakespeare: The Complete Works. New York, Barnes & Noble, 1994.

References

Adler J: Did Falstaff have the sleep-apnea syndrome? N Engl J Med 1983;308:404.

Andreasen NJ: The artist as scientist. Psychiatric diagnosis in Shakespeare's tragedies. JAMA 1976;235:1868–1872.

Anstey KJ, Low LF: Normal cognitive changes in aging. Aust Fam Physician 2004;33:783–787.

Donnelly J: Incest, ingratitude and insanity; aspects of the psychopathology of King Lear. Psychoanal Rev 1953;40:149–155.

Edgar II: Amariah Brigham, Isaac Ray and Shakespeare. Psychiatr Q 1961;35:666–674.

Fogan L: The neurology in Shakespeare. Arch Neurol 1989;46:922–924.

Furman Y, Wolf SM, Rosenfeld DS: Shakespeare and sleep disorders. Neurology 1997;49:1171–1172.

Hawley KS, Cherry KE, Su LJ, Chiu YW, Jazwinski SM: Knowledge of memory aging in adulthood. Int J Aging Hum Dev 2006;63:317–334.

Kail AC: The bard and the body. 1. Shakespeare's physicians. Med J Aust 1983;2:338–344.

Kail AC: The Medical Mind of Shakespeare. Balgowlah, Williams & Wilkins, 1986.

Kail AC: The doctors in Shakespeare's plays. Part two. Aust Fam Physician 1990;19:372–373, 376–378.

McKeith IG, Dickson DW, Lowe J, Emre M, O'Brien JT, Feldman H, Cummings J, Duda JE, Lippa C, Perry EK, Aarsland D, Arai H, Ballard CG, Boeve B, Burn DJ, Costa D, Del Ser T, Dubois B, Galasko D, Gauthier S, Goetz CG, Gomez-Tortosa E, Halliday G, Hansen LA, Hardy J, Iwatsubo T, Kalaria RN, Kaufer D, Kenny RA, Korczyn A, Kosaka K, Lee VM, Lees A, Litvan I, Londos E, Lopez OL, Minoshima S, Mizuno Y, Molina JA, Mukaetova-Ladinska EB, Pasquier F, Perry RH, Schulz JB, Trojanowski JQ, Yamada M; Consortium on DLB. Diagnosis and management of dementia with Lewy bodies: third report of the DLB Consortium. Neurology 2005;65:1863–1872.

Murray C: The People Who Matter II: The Giants; in Murray C: Human Accomplishment. New York, Harper Collins, 2003. pp 119–154.

Norton SA, Paris RM, Wonderlich KJ: 'Strange things I have in head': evidence of prion disease in Shakespeare's Macbeth. Clin Infect Dis 2006;42:299–302.

Peacock WG: Bedlam beggars, Winchester geese, and mewling infants: medicine and women's health issues in Shakespeare: presidential address. Am J Obstet Gynecol 2002;186:1196–1201.

Stien R: Shakespeare on parkinsonism. Mov Disord 2005;20:768–769.

Truskinovsky AM: Literary psychiatric observation and diagnosis through the ages: King Lear revisited. South Med J 2002;95:343–352.

Brandy R. Matthews, MD
Indiana University Neurology Outpatient Clinic
550 University Blvd UH 1710
Indianapolis, IN 46202 (USA)
Tel. +1 317 944 4000, Fax +1 317 278 2775, E-Mail brmatthe@iupui.edu

Bogousslavsky J, Hennerici MG, Bäzner H, Bassetti C (eds): Neurological Disorders in Famous
Artists – Part 3. Front Neurol Neurosci. Basel, Karger, 2010, vol 27, pp 227–237

The Neurology of Literature

G.D. Perkin

Charing Cross Hospital, London, UK

Abstract

The confines of this chapter are necessarily arbitrary. Its limits are partly imposed by
the extent of my reading (all the references have been read in full!) and partly by the
restrictions of space – as a consequence of that restriction there are innumerable examples
which I have been unable to cover. I have concentrated, though not exclusively, on the literature of the 19th century. There is much neurology in the modern novel, but the accessibility afforded by the internet and other sources to accounts of neurological symptoms and
diseases allows a present-day author an access that can bypass personal experience. Of
greater interest are those descriptions of neurological disorders which coincided with, or
even ante-dated, their appearance in the medical literature. My reading has been in English,
but has extended to works translated from Spanish, French, German and Russian. I have
concentrated on a small group of neurological conditions whose descriptions are of particular interest in the depth of observation they display, a depth suggesting they have
stemmed from first-hand experience. They are grouped under the headings of cerebrovascular disease, syncopal attacks and epilepsy.

One of the delights that a physician experiences when reading literature is
to encounter descriptions of diseases whose accuracy can come only from some
form of personal experience. In some cases, that experience is the result of personal suffering, most famously, perhaps, in the case of Dostoyevsky's complex
partial seizures. In other instances, it appears that the author has sought out a
physician to provide the necessary detail. Kipling, for example, is said to have
consulted with William Gowers when writing of Tabes Dorsalis in 'Love-o'-
Women'. Finally, where the descriptions are so numerous, as, for example, in
the novels of Charles Dickens, one has to assume that they depend on remarkable powers of personal observation.

Some Strokes

Sir Leicester Dedlock

He fell down this morning, a handsome, stately gentleman, somewhat infirm, but of a fine presence, and with a well-filled face. He lies upon his bed, an aged man with sunken cheeks, the decrepit shadow of himself. His voice was rich and mellow and he had so long been thoroughly persuaded of the weight and impact to mankind of any word he said that his words really had come to sound as if there were something in them. But now he can only whisper, and what he whispers sounds like what it is – mere jumble and jargon [Dickens, 1853].

Sir Leicester Dedlock has had a stroke. It occurred not without warning. Shortly before the event: 'Mr Bucket soon detects an unusual slowness in his speech, with now and then a curious trouble in beginning, which occasions him to utter inarticulate sounds' [Dickens, 1853].

The subsequent stroke partly recovers: 'I have had a sudden and bad attack. Something that deadens, making an endeavour to pass one hand down one side, "and confuses", touching his lips' [Dickens, 1853].

Sir Leicester evidently has a hemiparesis, presumably right-sided if he was right handed. If that were the case Dickens' description of the combination of a right hemiplegia with aphasia antedates that of Hughlings Jackson by some 11 years [Jackson, 1864].

Cleopatra Skewton

Dickens writes of other individuals with speech disorders.

Cleopatra Skewton, in Dombey and Son [Dickens, 1848] is certainly dysarthric but also dysphasic. The onset of her problem suggests a cerebrovascular event.

Powerful remedies were resorted to; opinions given that she would rally from this shock, but would not survive another; and there she lay speechless, and staring at the ceiling for days; sometimes making inarticulate sounds in answer to such questions as did she know who were present, and the like: sometimes giving no reply either by sign or gesture, or in her unwinking eyes.

At length she began to recover consciousness, and in some degree the power of motion, though not yet of speech. One day the use of her right hand returned; and showing it to her maid who was in attendance on her, and appearing very uneasy in her mind, she made signs for a pencil and some paper …

After much painful scrawling and erasing, and putting in wrong characters, which seemed to tumble out of the pencil of their own accord, the old woman produced this document: 'Rose-coloured curtains.'…

'Now, my dearest Grangeby', said Mrs. Skewton, 'you must posively prom', she cut some of her words short, and cut out others altogether, 'come down very soon'. … 'Sterious wretch, who's he?' lisped Cleopatra. …

'My dearest Edith – Grangeby – it's most trordinry thing', said Cleopatra, pettishly, … 'I won't have visitors – really don't want visitors', she said; 'little repose – and all that sort of thing – is what I quire. No odious brutes must proach me till I've shaken off this numbness'; …

Prince Nicholas Bolkónsky

The stroke or strokes suffered by Prince Nicholas Bolkónsky in Tolstoy's *War and Peace* (Tolstoy 1868–1869) are more complex affairs. It has been suggested that the initial episode is an example of the one-and-a-half syndrome [Albin, 1990]. The initial description establishes that the prince had had a 'seizure paralyzing his right side'. He is described as remaining unconscious for the next three weeks, though Princess Mary believes that his agitation in her presence suggested an awareness of her. Later he asks for her.

> He was lying on his back propped up high and his small bony hands with their knotted purple veins were lying on the quilt; his left eye gazed straight before him, his right eye was awry and his brows and lips motionless. … when she changed her position so that his left eye could see her face he calmed down, not taking his eyes off her for some seconds.

There is some paradox here. The suggestion that he kept his eyes on her for some seconds suggests that at that point, there was no squint. Furthermore, the suggestion that Princess Mary needed to move centrally either suggests Tolstoy is confusing the effects of an oculomotor paresis with a visual field defect, or that the Prince, in addition to his oculomotor disorder, had an homonymous defect to one or the other side. In addition he has a speech defect which Albin has suggested was dysarthric. I am less confident that is the correct description. 'He said something, repeating the same words several times. She could not understand them, but tried to guess what he was saying and inquiringly repeated the words he uttered.' Surprisingly, soon afterwards, and shortly before his second and fatal stroke, his speech appears to become coherent, both in terms of content and pronunciation.

Madam Raquin and M. Noirtier

Thérèse Raquin was published in 1867 [Zola, 1867]. Madame Raquin has a sudden event though it had been preceded by a gradually progressing paralysis.

> The poor old soul was beginning to mutter disconnected phrases, her voice was failing, and her limbs one after another were becoming useless … She did not notice the implacable paralysis which in spite of everything was making her stiffer day by day. On the fateful evening, she stopped in the middle of a sentence, open-mouthed, gaping, feeling as if she were being strangled. She tried to shout for help but could only utter raucous sounds. Her tongue had turned to stone. Her hands and feet had stiffened. She was struck dumb and motionless. … Then they realized that there was nothing left facing them but a body, a body half alive who could see and hear them but could not speak.
> That shapeless, pallid face … was like the decomposing mask of a dead woman with two living eyes set in it, and the eyes alone moved and turned quickly in their sockets, while the cheeks and mouth were petrified and set in a frightening stillness.

The condition has been diagnosed as a locked-in syndrome [Thompson and Martin, 1984], though the onset is atypical in that – 'for a few days Madame

Raquin kept the use of her hands and could write on a slate and ask for what she wanted; but then her hands went dead too.'

It is suggested that Thérèse, Madame Raquin's niece, was the only one who knew how to communicate with her aunt, though it is never made clear in the novel which eye movements are preserved and whether it is by that means that communication existed. Madame Raquin briefly regains partial use of her right hand and attempts, by spelling out the letters, to denounce her niece, whose lover has killed Madame Raquin's son, Camille.

A more detailed account of a locked-in syndrome was given by Alexandre Dumas in the Count of Monte Cristo, published over 20 years previously [Dumas, 1844–1846].

M. Noirtier, although almost as immovable and helpless as a corpse, looked at the newcomers with a quick and intelligent expression, perceiving at once, by their ceremonious courtesy, that they were come on business of an unexpected and official character. Sight and hearing were the only senses remaining and they appeared left, like two solitary sparks, to animate the miserable body which seemed fit for nothing but the grave; ... Valentine, by means of her love, her patience, and her devotion, had learned to read in Noirtier's look all the varied feelings which were passing in his mind. ...

It had been agreed that the old man should express his approbation by closing his eyes, his refusal by winking them several times, and, if he had some desire or feeling to express, he raised them to heaven. If he wanted Valentine, he closed the right eye only; and if Barrois, the left. ...

'Well sir, by the help of two signs, with which I will acquaint you presently, you may ascertain with perfect certainty that my grandfather is still in the full possession of all his mental faculties. M. Noirtier, being deprived of voice and motion, is accustomed to convey his meaning by closing his eyes when he wishes to signify "yes" and to wink when he means "no".'

This is a near perfect description of the locked-in syndrome, though the presence of independent winking of either eye suggests that there is some retention of facial nerve function.

The same novel contains another interesting neurological case, though I have been unable to identify it.

Now that I am safely here, let me explain to you the nature of my attack, and the appearance it will present. I am seized with a fit of catalepsy[1]; when it comes to its height, I may probably lie still and motionless as though dead, uttering neither sigh nor groan. On the other hand, the symptoms may be much more violent and cause me to fall into fearful convulsions, cover my lips with foaming, and force from me the most piercing shrieks. ...

'The former of these fits', said he, 'lasted but half an hour. At the termination of which I experienced no other feeling than a great sensation of hunger; and I rose from my bed without requiring the least help. Now I can neither move my right arm nor leg, and my head seems uncomfortable, proving a rush of blood in the brain. ...

[1] A favorite condition of 19th century novelists.

'Since the first attack I experienced of this malady I have continually reflected on it. Indeed, I expected it, for it is a family inheritance; both my father and grandfather having been taken off by it.'

The condition is genetically determined, and inherited as an autosomal dominant. Though the description of the attacks is somewhat bizarre, it can be assumed that some are epileptic, and apparently potentially followed by a hemiplegia. Are we dealing with familial cavernomas?

Syncopal Attacks

Cotton and Lewis [1918–1920], in their classical description of faints, concluded that 'accurate observations upon the cardiovascular system during the faints of which young men and women of nervous disposition are the subjects have not as yet been obtained, or obtained, have not been recorded'.

That comment rather ignored the previous observations of Gowers [1893], and certainly those in the literature of the previous two centuries.

I moved towards the Superior with my arms held out in supplication and my body leaning backwards, swooning. I fell, but it was not a heavy fall. In such fainting fits when one's strength abandons one, the limbs seem to give way and as it were fold up unawares; nature unable to hold up, seems to try to collapse gently. I lost consciousness and the sense of feeling and merely heard confused and distant voices buzzing round me; whether it was real speech or a singing in my ears, I could make out nothing but this continual buzzing [Diderot, 1780–1781].

Diderot emphasizes the gradual rather than precipitate fall of a faint, and the twilight state during recovery when external stimuli are deadened or distorted. Pallor, as an accompanying feature of the attack, was recognized by Jane Austen and George Eliot.

Marianne, now looking dreadfully white, and unable to stand, sunk on to her chair, and Elinor, expecting every moment to see her faint, tried to screen her from the observation of others, while reviving her with lavender water [Austin, 1811].

'Look there! She's fainting', said the landlady, hastening to support Hetty, who had lost her miserable consciousness and looked like a beautiful corpse [Eliot, 1859].

Other manifestations of the presyncopal state include blurring of vision, dimming or echoing of hearing and a slowing of responsiveness.

She staggered desperately, a few paces further and reached the first row of doors that opened on the landing. There nature sank exhausted: her knees gave way under her – her breath, her sight, her hearing all seemed to fail her together at the same instant – and she dropped down senseless on the floor at the head of the stairs [Collins, 1856–1857].

In his novels Dickens describes no fewer than 20 faints, or swoons (he used the terms interchangeably). All but one occurs in women and the exception, in Oliver Twist, is not typical since the swooning individual has, the previous day: '... twined his hands in his hair; and with a loud scream, rolled grovelling upon the floor, his eyes fixed, and the foam covering his lips' [Dickens, 1837–1839].

Dickens is surprisingly cursory in his description of the physical features of fainting. Miss Havedale is described as being very pale [Dickens, 1841], and Marleena, in Nicholas Nickleby confusingly reported: '... to fall stiff and rigid' [Dickens, 1839].

Dickens' fainters fall into two categories. The first are young women, generally responding to an emotional crisis rather than a physical insult. The second group can only be described as manipulative:

… at length Marleena (who quite forgot she had fainted, when she found she was not noticed) [Dickens, 1839].

Miss Petowker was at length supported in a condition of such exhaustion to the first floor, where she no sooner encountered the youthful bridegroom than she fainted with great decorum [Dickens, 1839].

Few other authors have been quite so direct in their recognition of an ulterior motive in so-called faints, though Trollope considered the possibility.

She pressed one hand against her heart, gasped for breath and then fell back upon the sofa. Perhaps she could have done nothing better. Had the fainting been counterfeit, the measure would have shown ability. But the fainting was altogether true [Trollope, 1873].

Though emotional factors are important in the genesis of faints, the sight of blood or a physical injury, are equally potent.

This was no other than the charming Sophia herself who from the sight of blood, or from fear of her father, or from other reason, had fallen down in a swoon, before anyone could get to her assistance [Fielding, 1749].

Emotional and physical factors can interact to the point where the witnessing of one faint leads to another.

So Bovary sent for a bandage and basin, which he asked Justin to hold
'Don't be afraid, my man' he said to the already white-faced villager.
'No, no, go ahead!' the man answered. And he held out his brawny arm with a touch of bravado. At the prick of the lancet the blood spurted out and splashed against the mirror.
'Nearer with the basin!' Charles exclaimed. 'Lookee!' said the peasant. 'It's like a young fountain flowing! What red blood I've got. Should be a good sign, eh?'
'Sometimes', the Officer of Health remarked, 'they don't feel anything at first: the syncope occurs afterwards, especially with strong chaps like this.'
Instantly the yokel let go of the lancet-case which he had been twirling in his fingers: a jerk of his shoulders snapped the back of his chair: his cap fell to the floor.
'I thought as much,' said Bovary, putting his fingers over the vein.
The basin began to wobble in Justin's hands. He quaked at the knees. His face went white.
'Emma!' Charles called out, 'Emma!' She was down the stairs in a flash. 'Vinegar!' he cried. 'Good Lord, two at once!' [Flaubert, 1856–1857].

Vinegar figures prominently in literature as an efficacious remedy, as does water. Elizabeth Gaskell recognized the importance of posture in aiding recovery from a faint.

'Give me the water. Run for Mama, Mary' said Jemima, as she saw that the fainting fit did not yield to the usual remedy of a horizontal position and the water- sprinkling [Gaskell, 1853].

Arnold Bennett recognized the danger of trying to support the fainting individual.

'Never raise the head of a person who has lost consciousness', he said coldly, 'it is dangerous. Teresa will recover in a few minutes. This swoon is due only to the shock and strain of the last few minutes' [Bennett, 1931].

There are other conditions causing loss of consciousness which can masquerade as faints. Syncope arising from a cardiac arrhythmia is not confined to the elderly.

'By jove, what a rate my heart is galloping at! These confounded palpitations get worse instead of better'....

Still he might only have fainted; it might only be a fit. Sir Christopher knelt down, unfastened the cravat, unfastened the waistcoat, and laid his hand on the heart. It might be syncope; it might not – it could not be death. No! That thought must be kept far off [Eliot, 1858].

Epilepsy

In recent times, misconceptions regarding epilepsy and those who suffer from the condition have lessened. Many of these misconceptions abound in literature, particularly from the 19th century, though they are matched in the neurological writings of that century. Romberg and Gowers stressed the epileptic temperament and the inevitable intellectual decline of those with the condition. Physical appearance was thought to declare the condition, an opinion shared by Dostoyevsky.

Something of that strange expression which makes people realize at the first glance that they are dealing with an epileptic [Dostoyevsky, 1868–1869].

Both neurologists and novelists of the 19th century emphasized the epileptic cry.

… uttering a piercing cry that alarms both mankind and animals [Romberg, 1853].

He twisted his hands in his hair, and with a loud scream, rolled grovelling upon the floor, his eyes fixed, and the foam covering his lips [Dickens, 1837–1839].

Dostoyevsky emphasized the phenomenon based on personal knowledge. A witness to one of his fits described a peculiar, prolonged and meaningless cry at the onset of a seizure [Pierce Clark, 1915]. The cry figures recurringly in the seizures suffered by his characters.

She did not see the fall, but heard his scream – the strange, peculiar scream she had long known, the scream of the epileptic falling in a fit [Dostoyevsky, 1880].

Prince Mischkin suffers similarly: the first sound of the dreadful scream, which burst from his chest of its own accord and which he could have done nothing to suppress [Dostoyevsky, 1868–1869].

Dostoyevsky had complex partial seizures, recognizing the onset of an attack before he lost consciousness, and describing those prodromal symptoms in some of his characters.

There are seconds – they come five or six at a time – when you suddenly feel the presence of eternal harmony in all its fullness. It is nothing earthly. I don't mean that it is heavenly, but a man in his earthly semblance can't endure it. He has to undergo a physical change or die. … in those five seconds I live through a lifetime, and I am ready to give my life for them, for it's worth it. …

'Kirilov, does this often happen?'

'Once in three days, once a week.'

'You're not an epileptic?'

'No.'

'You will be one. Take care, Kirilov. I've heard that's just how an epileptic fit begins. An epileptic described to me exactly that preliminary sensation before a fit, exactly as you've done' [Dostoyevsky, 1871].

Dostoyevsky assumed that all attacks had a prodroma.

It is, of course, impossible to foretell the day or hour of such attacks, but every epileptic can feel beforehand that he is liable to have such an attack. That is the opinion of the medical profession [Dostoyevsky, 1880].

Accounts of the physical changes accompanying a seizure are numerous. Elizabeth Gaskell refers to the cyanosis [Gaskell, 1863–1864] and Thomas Mann to the physical contortions.

… and one day, while the meal was in full swing, the man was seized with a violent epileptic fit, and with that oft-described demoniac unearthly shriek fell to the floor, where he lay beside this chair striking about him with dreadfully distorted arms and legs [Mann, 1924].

Short-lived neurological signs following a seizure have the same significance as an aura – they suggest a focal basis for the event.

He spoke to them in something of his own voice too, but sharpened and made hollow like a dead man's face. What he would have said, God knows. He seemed to utter words, but they were such as man had never heard. And this was the most fearful circumstance of all, to see him standing there, gabbling in an unearthly tongue [Dickens, 1844].

Anthony Chuzzlewit is dysphasic after his seizure and dies soon afterwards.

Seizures in childhood are unlikely to produce persisting focal deficit unless the consequence of a middle cerebral or internal carotid occlusion, when they will be accompanied by a persistent hemiplegia.

You see, my poor child, I and my sister Cora are a great deal older than you and we both had convulsions when we were about your age. You may have noticed that our left arms are rather stiff and our left legs, too [Peake, 1946].

The twin sisters, who appear to have learning difficulties, appear confused about which side of their body is affected. Later they refer to being practically starved all down the right side and later still, imply both sides of the body have suffered.

'Not only our left arms', Clarice broke in, 'but all down our left-hand sides and our right-hand legs, too' [Peake, 1946].

Complex partial seizures, by their very nature, pose much greater diagnostic challenges than do tonic-clonic seizures. Part of the challenge arises from the fact that certain phenomena, for example déjà-vu, are a part of everyday experience.

We have all some experience of a feeling that comes over us occasionally, of what we are saying and doing having been said and done before, in a remote time. Of our having been surrounded, dim ages ago, by the same faces, objects and circumstances – of our knowing perfectly what will be said next, as if we suddenly remembered it! [Dickens, 1850].

The reaction is triggered in David Copperfield by a remark of Mr Micawber's, suggesting a confusion in Copperfield's mind between his affection for Dora, his wife, and Agnes Wickfield.

Beyond this are more complex sensations which, though often ascribed by the writer to a mystic experience, have characteristics more supportive of epilepsy.

Once more the scent of pinks came quivering through his brain and he felt a nameless twirl of pleasure. This time, instead of the wraith of Christie Malakite, it was the body of the hatter that associated itself with that remembered scent – not any repulsive odour of mortality emerging from those nailed-up boards, but rather some spiritual essence from the presence of Death itself. And as he breathed this air, the voices of his companions became a vague humming in his ears, and all manner of queer detached memories floated in upon him. He felt himself to be walking alone along some high white road bordered by waving grasses and patches of yellow rock-rose. There was a town far below him, at the bottom of a green valley – a mass of huddled grey roofs among meadows and stream – round which the twilight was darkening. Along with all this he was conscious of the taste of a peculiar kind of baker's bread, such as used to be sold at a shop in Dorchester, where as a child, they would take him for tea during summer jaunts from Weymouth [Powys, 1929].

Non-organic epileptic seizures may occur at a conscious or subconscious level. I have not encountered examples of the latter in literature, but several of the former. Felix Krull simulates epilepsy to avoid military service. In his interview in the recruiting office he develops periodic jerking and twitching of the shoulders. Later he indicates that a particular indisposition prevented him from completing the 7th grade at school. Krull suggests that the family doctor diagnosed the problem as migraine but then announces to the interviewing panel 'a great feeling of distress and fear'. Finally the seizure appears.

My face became contorted … my features were literally thrust apart in all directions … my head lolled and several times it twisted almost entirely around just as if Old Nick were in the act of breaking my neck; my shoulders and arms seemed at the point of being wrenched out of their sockets, my hips were bowed, my knees turned inward, my belly was hollowed, while my ribs seemed to burst the skin over them; my teeth were clamped together, not a single finger but was fantastically bent into a claw [Mann, 1954].

The doctor on the board is taken in.

'This person summoned for duty', he explained in a thin bleat 'suffers from epileptoid attacks, the so-called equivalents which are sufficient to negate absolutely his fitness for service … the appearance of the so-called aura was unmistakable in the patient's obviously embarrassed description.' It is worth noting that even today, there persists in the consciousness of many epileptics something of that mystical, religious attitude which the ancient world adopted towards this nervous disorder.

References

Albin RA: The death of Nicholas Bolkónski. Neurology in Tolstoy's War and Peace. Arch Neurol 1990;47:225–226.
Austin J: Sense and Sensibility, Whitehall, T. Edgerton, 1811.
Bennett A: Terese of Watling Street. London, Ward Lock & Co. 1931.
Collins W: The Dead Secret. London, Household Words, 1856–1857.
Cotton TF, Lewis T: Observation upon fainting attacks due to inhibitory cardiac impulses. Heart 1918–1920;7:23–34.
Dickens C: Oliver Twist. London, Richard Bentley, 1837–1839.
Dickens C: Nicholas Nickelby. London, Chapman & Hall, 1839.
Dickens C: Barnaby Rudge. London, Chapman & Hall, 1841.
Dickens C: Martin Chuzzlewit. London, Chapman & Hall, 1844.
Dickens C: Dombey and Son. London, Bradbury & Evans, 1848.
Dickens C: David Copperfield. London, Bradbury & Evans, 1850.
Dickens C: Bleak House. London, Bradbury & Evans, 1853.
Diderot D: The Nun. Paris, Correspondance Littéraire, 1780–1781.
Dostoyevsky F: The Idiot. Moscow, Rússkii Véstnik, 1868–1869.
Dostoyevsky F: The Devils. Moscow, Rússkii Véstnik, 1871.
Dostoyevsky F: The Brothers Karamazov. Moscow, Rússkii Véstnik, 1880.
Dumas A: The Count of Monte Cristo. Paris, Pétion, 1844–1846.
Eliot G: Scenes of Clerical Life. Edinburgh, William Blackwood, 1858.
Eliot G: Adam Bede. Edinburgh, William Blackwood, 1859.
Fielding H: Tom Jones. London, A. Millar, 1749.
Flaubert G: Madame Bovary. Paris, Revue de Paris, 1856–1857.
Gaskell E: Ruth. London, Chapman & Hall, 1853.
Gaskell E: Cousin Phillis. London, Cornhill Magazine, 1863–1864.
Gowers WR: A Manual of Diseases of the Nervous System, ed 2. London, J & A Churchill, 1893.
Jackson HJ: Hemiplegia on the right side with loss of speech. Br Med J 1864;i:572.
Mann T: The Magic Mountain. Berlin, S. Fischer, 1924.
Mann T: Confessions of Felix Krull, Confidence Man. Berlin, S. Fischer, 1954.
Peake M: Titus Groan. London, Eyre & Spottiswoode,1946.
Pierce Clark L: A study of the epilepsy of Dostojewsky. Boston Med Surg J 1915;169:1–18.
Powys JC: Wolf Solent. New York, Simon & Schuster, 1929.

Romberg MH: A Manual of the Nervous Diseases of Man. Translated and edited by Sievéking EH. London, Sydenham Society, 1853.
Thompson AJ, Martin EA: Zola and the 'locked-in' syndrome. Neurology 1984;34:1212.
Tolstoy L: War and Peace. Moscow, Rússkii Véstnik, 1868–1869.
Trollope A: The Eustace Diamonds. London, Chapman & Hall, 1873.
Zola E: Thérèse Raquin. Paris, Lacroix, 1867.

Dr. G.D. Perkin
Charing Cross Hospital
Fulham Palace Road
London, W6 8RF (UK)
Tel. +44 208 846 1184, Fax +44 208 846 7487, E-Mail d.perkin@ic.ac.uk

....

Author Index

Subject Index